"*Accessible Ashtanga* is a book that I never expected to see in my lifeti the power of the yoga teachings to continue to expand like waves in ᵁ.ᵁ ᵁᵁᵁᵁᵁ ᵁᵁᵁ every shore, touching the lives of people of all abilities all over the world. After all, yoga's fundamental teaching is that we all share the same heart, so how can we practice the fullness of yoga without recognizing that it needs to be adapted to reach everyone? I applaud Kino MacGregor's bravery for jumping into the ocean of accessibility and throwing us a lifeline. Her insights are simultaneously new and traditional, which is a balance that only a masterful teacher can find. The call to share yoga with all is not a simple one—especially for teachers of specific yoga traditions. As Kino explains, 'When the rules stop working for you, it's time to either change or break the rules. The ability to adapt the series and poses to better fit a diversity of students is the hallmark of this special moment we are in right now.'"

—Jivana Heyman, author of *The Teacher's Guide to Accessible Yoga*

"Thank you, Kino, for providing a valuable resource for both Ashtanga enthusiasts of all levels as well as lovers of yoga from other disciplines to feel welcome and encouraged to pursue their unique path and personal expression of practice. With a multitude of photos, clear instructions, inspiring quotes, and philosophical insights, your presentation is a welcome contribution to the rich heritage of yoga."

—David Swenson, author of *Ashtanga Yoga*

"*Accessible Ashtanga* is a must-read for students brand new to yoga, as well as long time practitioners. It reveals the deep therapeutic and contemplative potential of the Ashtanga Vinyasa practice, where the breath, feelings, emotions, and all thought patterns are treated as interwoven and sacred. Kino's direct and clear teachings put Ashtanga within reach for anyone wanting to experience the joys and benefits of a personal practice that supports daily life."

—Richard Freeman and Mary Taylor, authors of *When Love Comes to Light*

"In *Accessible Ashtanga*, Kino MacGregor tackles a task many might think of as impossible: sharing the primary series in a way that connects to more bodies and experiences while preserving the depth of the practice. She provides solid foundations, and then she gives us many variations and options for practice. While there is never going to be one definitive way to create accessibility, Kino gives us many different options and provides us with clear, informative examples to deepen our understanding and practice. I'm thrilled that in *Accessible Ashtanga* we have a guidebook for how to practice and teach the primary series in a more accessible, heartfelt, and connected way."

—Susanna Barkataki, author of *Embrace Yoga's Roots*

"*Accessible Ashtanga* is a book everyone will benefit from—a thought-provoking, revolutionary, and innovative approach to the Ashtanga practice. While still maintaining her firm belief in the tradition, Kino MacGregor challenges the popular discourse of modern yoga, which correlates physical ability with spiritual progress. Instead, Kino offers practical techniques, creative advice, and invaluable wisdom with which to create and foster a more inclusive space for all!"

—David Robson and Jelena Vesić, yoga teachers

ACCESSIBLE
ASHTANGA

An All-Levels Guide to the
Primary and Intermediate Series

Kino MacGregor

Foreword by Shanna Small

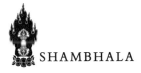

SHAMBHALA

Shambhala Publications, Inc.
2129 13th Street
Boulder, Colorado 80302
www.shambhala.com

Photographs by Yoandy Vidal and Osmani Tellez

Cover photo: Yoandy Vidal and Osmani Tellez
Cover design: Daniel Urban-Brown
Interior design: Laura Shaw Design

9 8 7 6 5 4 3 2 1

First Edition
Printed in the United States of America

Shambhala Publications makes every effort to print on
acid-free, recycled paper.
Shambhala Publications is distributed worldwide
by Penguin Random House, Inc., and its subsidiaries.

Library of Congress Cataloging-in-Publication Data

Names: MacGregor, Kino, author. | Small, Shanna, author of foreword.
Title: Accessible Ashtanga: an all-levels guide to the primary and intermediate
series / Kino MacGregor; foreword by Shanna Small.
Description: First edition. | Boulder, Colorado: Shambhala, [2024] |
Identifiers: LCCN 2023029190 | ISBN 9781645470816 (trade paperback)
Subjects: LCSH: Aṣṭāṅga yoga.
Classification: LCC RA781.68 .M3198 2024 | DDC 613.7/046—dc23/
eng/20231208
LC record available at https://lccn.loc.gov/2023029190

Contents

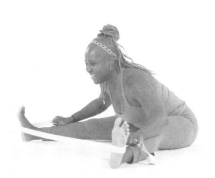
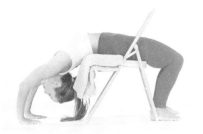
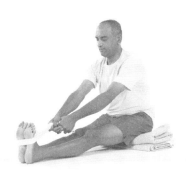

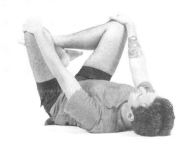

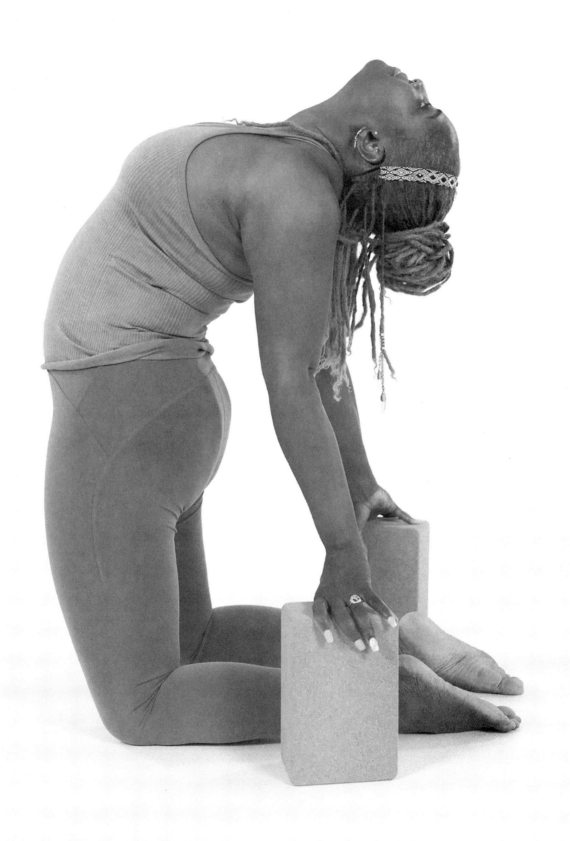

Foreword

THE PURPOSE OF YOGA is repeated throughout the tradition's texts and traditions: freedom from the never-ending cycle of pain and suffering. So, in theory, liberation should be the common goal and at the center of all yoga. But liberation can never look the same for everyone because we are all bound by different shackles. There are emotional shackles such as shame, vanity, anger, greed, and envy. There are physical shackles that show up as disease in the body. There are shackles we share with the community that are systemic, such as racism, sexism, and ableism. There are shackles that are passed down through our DNA as family trauma. The impediments and obstacles that bind us determine at least in part how our yoga will look and what techniques we will need for our liberation.

The route to freedom and liberation must be appropriate for the individual. In yoga, the student needs the proper tools and instructions that work with their "vehicle"—their body—and the operating system of the mind. Traditionally, yoga was student-centered, thereby making it inherently accessible. Students were taught individually or in small groups by a teacher. Unfortunately, yoga has been colonized, corporatized, and commodified into a practice that is now taught in large groups with a specific body ideal in mind.

When taught in its traditional Mysore style, Ashtanga Yoga is inherently accessible. In Mysore-style Ashtanga, students learn pose by pose with a teacher. The student is given pose variations based on their body and life circumstances. Guided classes are introduced after the student knows what to do with their own body. When students attend a guided class, they do their variations and then sit and watch when they get to parts of the practice they have not yet learned.

While many teachers and students still approach Ashtanga this way, the media shows a different picture. Society often uplifts the most complex versions of Ashtanga poses and the people who do them. Comparison, the thief of joy, is rampant in the Ashtanga community. Practice rooms are flooded with able-bodied people who want to look like the popular practitioners on social media, and teachers have shifted how they teach to meet this demand and to sell the dream. In order for Ashtanga to be accessible, we must remind ourselves of yoga's original purpose and shift our focus from the attainment of poses back to the attainment of liberation.

While the roots of Ashtanga are accessible, innovation is still necessary. For some, *innovation* is a bad word that is associated with appropriation. Appropriation is stealing yoga and commodifying it, all while not honoring the source culture. However, there has always been room for innovation in yoga. Traditionally, yoga is passed down from teacher to student. Every iteration keeps its roots while adding a dash of modernity so the practice is appropriate for the students of the time. That is innovation. Traditionally, Ashtanga has not used props such as blocks, straps, and chairs; however, it is an innovation that can make Ashtanga more accessible.

Without the chair, I would have stopped practicing Ashtanga years ago. A few years ago, I fell down a flight of stairs and sprained ligaments that supported the left side of my sacrum and hip. After many trips to the doctor, I also discovered that my disc at L5, the base of my spine, was eroded and that my sacrum was fused with that disc on the left side. I had arthritis and pinched nerves that resulted in debilitating pain and trouble walking. I had been practicing Ashtanga for close to twenty years, and I loved my practice. However, it was impossible for me to practice without pain. I took a training that taught me about variations and how to use chairs. Using the chair allowed me to continue my Ashtanga practice without pain while my body continued to heal. When I started to feel better, I moved to props such as blocks, bolsters, and blankets. I continue to use props today to deal with the lingering effects of my accident.

Variations, chairs, and other props are not only to accommodate injury. While I was going through my healing process, I learned about hypermobility and how most bodies stay at "functional range"—a medical term that refers to the range of motion required to maintain independence for daily activities. Most bodies only move within functional range. Hypermobile joints move outside of that range. Most yoga poses, offered in a typical group class, are outside of functional range. This means that most people have bodies that can't do yoga without pose variations. Why then are most of the students in yoga classes hypermobile? Because modern yoga classes are self-selecting. Because the commodification of yoga means more standardized classes where hypermobile people tend to stick around. Folks at functional range are few and far between and don't tend to stay for the long run. Why would they? They are being presented with a practice that goes far beyond what their bodies will ever be able to do.

This takes us back to the original purpose of yoga and how everyone is worthy of liberation. I have not seen any proof that hypermobility and liberation go hand and hand. On the contrary, hypermobility, when overexploited, can lead to pain, which is the opposite of freedom and liberation. The use of props equalizes access to this liberatory practice of Ashtanga Yoga and makes it accessible to all bodies. There is a prevalent myth in the world of yoga that hard work can overcome all bodily concerns, but genetics say otherwise. Add the daily unique stressors of life and unexpected accidents and events, and it quickly becomes apparent that every body is not the same.

The biggest obstacle to making Ashtanga accessible is a closed mind and a system that touts and profits off the belief that all bodies are inherently the same. Yoga is for everyone; accessibility is the only way for everyone to tap into its healing power. For yoga to be accessible, we must embrace its student-centered roots. Every person who shows up for class is worthy of liberation and the healing power of yoga.

—SHANNA SMALL

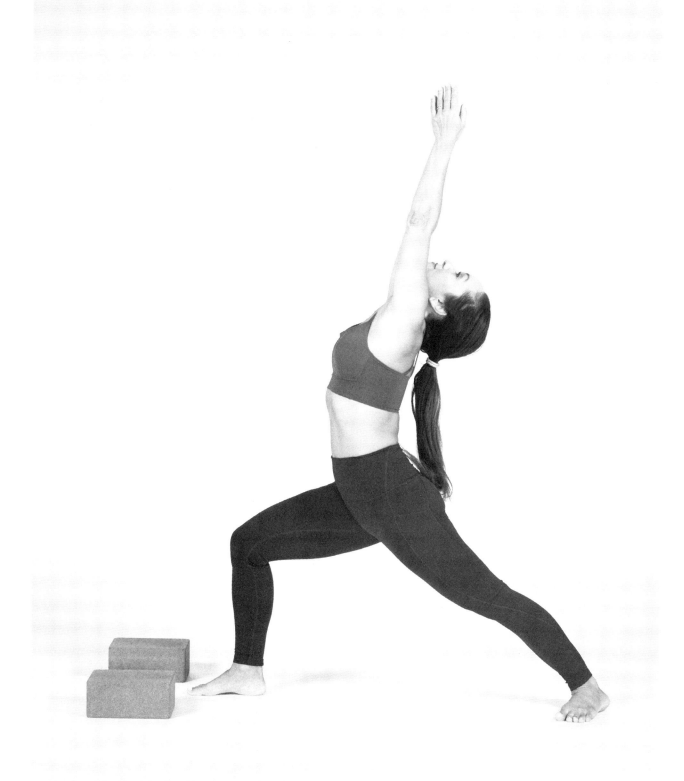

Acknowledgments

WITH LOVE AND RESPECT to my mom, whose fiery spirit, tenacity, and double total knee replacement inspired my journey into accessibility.

Special thanks to Lashanna Small for contributing the foreword and for her leadership in the Ashtanga community, to Monica Arellano for her extensive help compiling and organizing all the photos and for her appearance in many of the asanas in this book, to Yoandy Vidal and Osmani Tellez for their amazing photography work throughout what sometimes felt like a never-ending photoshoot, and to Tatiana Uprimmy and the whole Omstars team for always having my back when it comes to bringing the message of yoga to the world.

Much gratitude to all the teachers who contributed their thoughtful quotes to this book: David Swenson, Hamish Hendry, Mary Taylor and Richard Freeman, Wambui Njuguna-Räisänen, Ajay Tokas, Ty Landrum, Kira Williams Bouwer, Marcos Silva, Meetali Meshram, Tim Feldmann, Taylor Hunt, Joseph Armstrong, and Dr. Pavithra Kumar. Your words, teachings, and contributions are respected and cherished.

In honor of Edgar Navarro, Umashankar Annapa, Eddy Rivero, and all the student and teacher models who authentically and honestly shared their practice to make this book possible.

In recognition of my publisher, Shambhala, and editor, Beth Frankl, whose belief in my teaching and my message has made this book and many others possible.

In humble appreciation to all the students of yoga, especially those who have practiced with me in person or online, have read my books, and are a part of the community of fellow seekers on the path of yoga. My work is in service to your practice, perseverance, and dedications.

As always, a deep *pranam* to my teachers, K. Pattabhi Jois and R. Sharath Jois, for their unwavering commitment to the traditional practice of Ashtanga Yoga.

ACCESSIBLE ASHTANGA

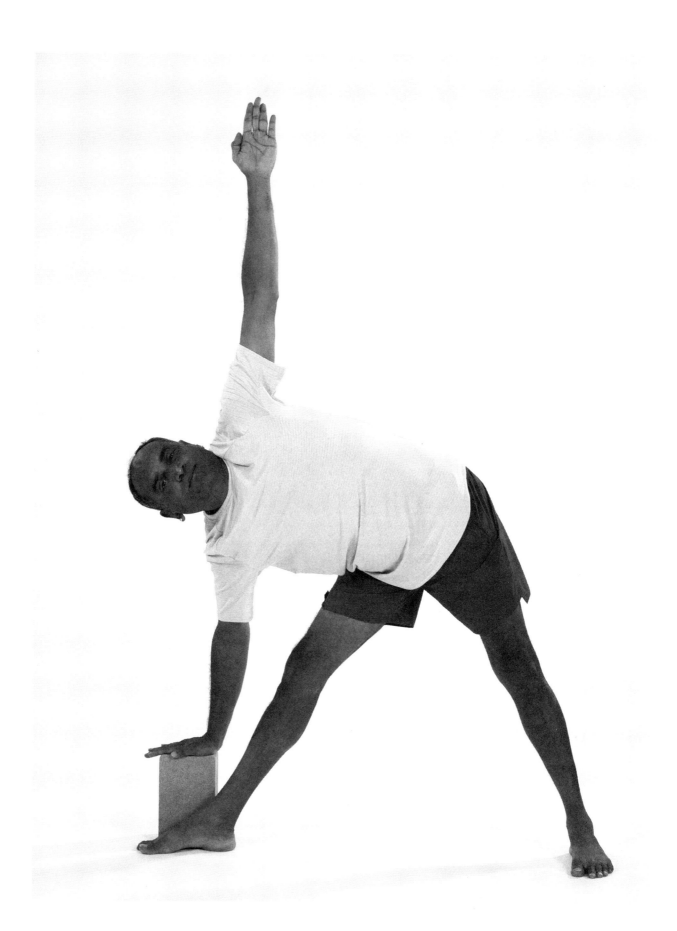

Introduction

ASHTANGA YOGA has a reputation for being hard and sometimes daunting. Beginners can feel easily overwhelmed and unsure if what they're doing is safe or not. Having a teacher's guidance helps students to avoid the pitfalls of injury, lack of confidence, or confusion. But not all teachers within the Ashtanga Yoga community know how to provide guidance to make the practice truly accessible to all. The purpose of this book is to give students and teachers the guidance needed to confidently adapt the practice of Ashtanga Yoga without losing the spiritual heart of the lineage. Having the tools to make the appropriate adjustments to the poses so they really work for every body is the key to taking this traditional practice to more inspired students all over the world.

While I have written two other Ashtanga Yoga books, this is by far the most challenging—not because there are *not enough* ways to adapt the poses but rather because there are *so many* ways to adapt the poses. The teachings in this book are the direct result of my more than twenty years of experience teaching real students the method of yoga that I learned from my teachers, R. Sharath Jois and K. Pattabhi Jois, in India. There was a time when variations and modifications were considered a kind of heresy. I believe that time has passed. In fact, I believe the future of Ashtanga Yoga is in adaptability. The asana needs to be adjusted so that its essence can best be used by each student. It is a difficult line to walk for the teacher, who has the responsibility to provide as many different variations as students show up to do the practice.

Whether you approach this book as a teacher looking for an accessible method of teaching or as a student seeking direction on adapting the practice, I hope you find a path forward through all the options presented here. However, by no means do I mean this to be the end of the exploration of asana. Instead, I hope this is the beginning of a new paradigm of thought within this lineage. I encourage you to find what works for yourself and expand on what I present here. My teaching is constantly evolving, and this is a snapshot of where I am today, in this moment. While the written word always appears codified, you make it come alive when you apply these teachings to yourself. So perhaps it is my intention for you, the reader, to be empowered to find your own voice and unique expression by standing on the firm ground of the research and experience I provide.

Some would argue that the very concept of accessible Ashtanga is a radical reconceptualization of this traditional lineage-based yoga practice. While it has been uncommon to modify the poses in the series in some more dogmatic approaches to the practice, I have always seen rules as rough guidelines rather than absolutes. When the rules stop working for you, it's time to either change or break the rules. The ability to adapt the series and poses to better fit a diversity of students is the hallmark of this special moment we are in right now. It could be seen as a kind of evolution of Ashtanga Yoga. Together, we are inviting the yoga practice to move beyond the dogmatic framework that sometimes appears in the traditional model. In this book, I intend to reframe the Ashtanga Yoga practice as something fresh and new and accessible to all while at the same time honoring the traditional teaching and lineage. I hope this book will be a valuable resource for teachers as well as offer a true, all-levels guide to the Ashtanga Yoga method.

Before we proceed, I must take a moment and acknowledge the work of Jivana Heyman, who is a true leader in the field of accessibility in yoga. Without his pioneering efforts to bring yoga to all people who desire the benefits of the practice, this book would not have been possible. Interspersed throughout this book you will find reflections on the Ashtanga lineage from a few key voices within the community. My intention has been to lift up and include different perspectives from teachers and students who are on the path of their personal practice. Seeing the true diversity of the community and hearing the different perspectives that they each share helps us see a fuller picture of what the living lineage looks like in this snapshot of time. As you read this book, reflect on what yoga means to you, ask the difficult questions of where you fit into the lineage and how you can best do the inner work of yoga in each practice and each day of your life.

Part One presents a new paradigm for yogic study in our contemporary age that deconstructs the guru model and decolonizes the yoga practice. A collection of comments and provoking thoughts from leaders in the Ashtanga Yoga community are included throughout this section.

Part Two presents each of the poses of the Ashtanga Yoga Primary Series and some of the poses of the Ashtanga Yoga Intermediate/Second Series in various forms for all levels. Not only will you see how to adapt the poses but you will learn how best to work the poses for your unique learning. Teachers will find a vast trove of reference material that will update their teaching methodology. Students will find adaptations that make the practice accessible and give their bodies permission to explore all sorts of options for practice. If you are brand new to the practice of Ashtanga Yoga, please do not attempt to practice the entire Primary and Intermediate/ Second Series in one shot. Ideally, seek the support of a qualified teacher to best assess which poses are right for your personal practice and then use the options presented here to supplement your work on the mat. If a qualified teacher is not available in person, then search for support online in videos, live classes, and other interactive modes of teaching where you can create the foundation of a personal practice through dialogue within the lineage. Along the way, this book will be a resource that will inform how you approach, adapt, and integrate the practice of Ashtanga Yoga to build a lifelong yoga sadhana.

Throughout the entire text, the spiritual journey of Ashtanga Yoga is kept as the main focus. While presenting a physical practice, I hope that you will be inspired to take the lessons you learn on the mat and translate them into spiritual life learning. In this presentation the spiritual journey only gets deeper and broader, like a wide path that makes space for all.

Everything that I present here rests firmly on the shoulders of my teachers, K. Pattabhi Jois and R. Sharath Jois, whose tireless dedication is the foundation of my personal practice. Placing Ashtanga Yoga within the contemporary world is not an easy task. I proceed intentionally with each step, weaving together the interdisciplinary faculties of feminism, antiracism, deconstructionism, and critical thinking. This book is a synthesis of the many spaces that I occupy within the yoga world, one part traditional and one part contemporary, one part critical and one part romantic. Without the myriad of students, colleagues, and collaborative voices who have each played a part in the evolution of Ashtanga Yoga, this book would not have come into being. It is not me but we who are making the change that we seek, together as one.

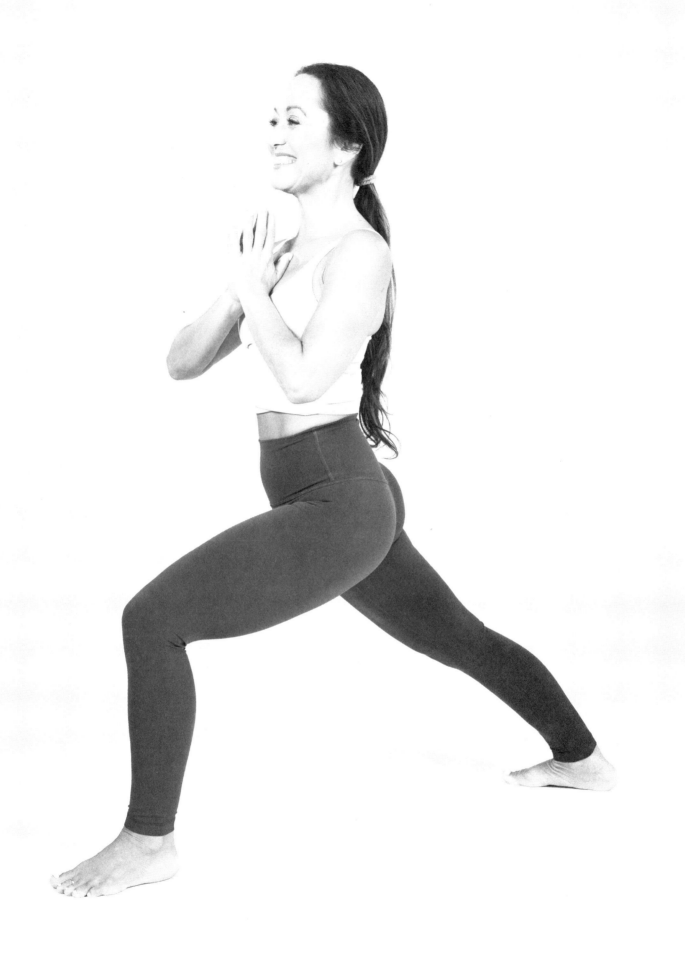

A New Paradigm

THERE IS A PROFOUND connection between the practice of yoga and the lives we live off the mat. Each breath and each sensation intricately reflect the depths of our selves, like a mirror that unveils the hidden habit patterns ingrained within. Yoga is a spiritual tool that empowers each practitioner to turn away from the potential for harm and nurture positivity. Gaining this sacred knowledge all depends on the attitude we bring to the mat. If we seek shortcuts, succumb to self-doubt, or strive for perfection, we deprive ourselves of the immeasurable benefits of the practice. But if we learn to devote ourselves with patience and perseverance, we can infuse every aspect of our lives with the healing power of yoga.

Yoga practice is not something that was invented in modern times. Yoga as a spiritual quest is a timeless tradition preserved for generations within India. Yet, at the same time, yoga practice in our modern era is unlike yoga practice at any other time in history. The practice is readily available to people all over the world, whether in person or online. The unprecedented juncture in which we find ourselves presents us with an opportunity to develop what may be considered a new paradigm of practice. There is a fine line between respecting the lineage and tradition of yoga and facing the realities of students and teachers alike, and I hope you will walk this path together with me.

1

Discovering the Real Meaning of the Ashtanga Method

THE TRADITIONAL DEFINITION of the Ashtanga method comes from Patanjali's Yoga Sutras. When we first approach the yoga mat with the intention to practice Ashtanga, the first thing Patanjali promises us is suffering. Don't stop reading, especially if you're new to the practice. It's not all or only about suffering. There is a light at the end of the tunnel.

While this might seem like an intense place to begin, there is great liberation in accepting, sitting with, and ultimately healing our pain. So much suffering has been created by false stories, stories that we tell ourselves about reality that create a spin divorced from the truth. We then take action based on those stories, and our actions lead to suffering. If we fail to understand how to approach our own suffering and the origin of our own suffering with kind hearts, then we might miss the whole opportunity of the journey of yoga.

The deeper purpose of Ashtanga Yoga is to burn through impurities of the mind, body, and spirit so we can seek and ultimately clearly perceive the truth about ourselves and the whole world. We use the practice to light the fire of purification, and the discomfort we feel in our bodies, in our minds, in our hearts' center, is the purifying fire through which we cleanse ourselves of bad habits and negative thoughts.

To be human is to suffer, and whether we realize it or not, we are defined by our suffering—or at least by how we respond to our suffering. *Suffering* is a word that could perhaps use a little context. Utilized as a key concept in both yoga methodology and the teaching of the Buddha, "suffering" comes from the Sanskrit word *dukha*. More than physical pain, dukha includes discomfort; feelings of unease; a general sense of malaise or dissatisfaction about the way things are, including craving, clinging, and ignorance. Dukha is a foundational concept within the wisdom traditions of the East, and the methodology of spiritual liberation is based on changing our

Ashtanga Yoga is a powerful tool that has far-reaching, deeply meaningful benefits to those that practice it. I do not say that Ashtanga is the best system or that it is for everyone, but I do believe it is for ANYONE. I have never met a person yet that cannot do Ashtanga Yoga. I have of course met folks that do not want to practice it, but that is another story. If someone is not interested, I do not try to change their opinion. I merely express that I enjoy it and then proceed to talk about other things. However, as teachers, it is our duty to find a way to present Ashtanga so that anyone expressing an interest may be given the chance to participate. We must facilitate practice for people of ALL shapes, sizes, ages, and physical abilities or lack thereof.

—DAVID SWENSON

habitual response to suffering and thereby destroying the ego. Old patterns rooted in ignorance create an endless cycle of suffering. If we spark the flame of awakening and walk through the fire—our own purification process—the cycle will not immediately come to a heroic and glorious end. We must endure while this flame burns through our impurities and wait for that same flame to light the lamp of knowledge. Along the way, the practice gives us the tools we need to overcome the obstacles set before us. This process is the Ashtanga method. It can take centuries of practice to reach enlightenment, but Ashtanga provides every student with exactly what they need to step and stay on the path. The practice influences everything from food to thoughts to speech to profession to relationships and family. The promise of Ashtanga Yoga is for all who practice with deep spiritual intention—that is, that if we persevere, we will eventually come out stronger on the other side. Suffering may not be eradicated entirely, but our response to the inevitable discomforts of life will be changed substantially for the better.

ALWAYS A STUDENT

Yoga is a journey, and at the heart of this journey is the student. Think back to your first yoga class. There is probably a bit of nostalgia around that memory. Or if you have not yet been to a yoga class, think about the butterflies in your stomach that arise when you contemplate unrolling your mat in a dedicated yoga space.

I'm a yoga teacher now, but I will always be a student. To be a student of yoga means the mind is open and inspired to learn, to practice. The quest of yoga is to find *nirodha*, the Sanskrit word defined as "stillness and inner peace." This inspiration is never stronger than at the very beginning of the journey. The concept of beginner's mind was first presented by the Zen Buddhist teacher Suzuki Roshi, and it is the perfect attitude to hold throughout the journey of yoga.

I will always remember my first yoga class, where it all began. I never had any intention of taking such a class. Not at first, anyway. When I was nineteen, I just happened to see a group of people at my gym standing on their heads. I thought to myself, "How amazing! I want to do that!" and signed up for my first class. It was a Hatha Yoga class, and I did not realize that joining it would forever alter the direction of my life. There was no standing on my head in that first class, but the impression of yoga as a spiritual practice was etched in my mind. While you might find this hard to believe now, I could not touch my toes in a simple forward fold. Instead of discouraging me from doing yoga, my lack of strength and flexibility inspired me to learn more. I found books and practiced at home until I found the Ashtanga Yoga lineage.

Then, when I was twenty-two years old, I joined a traditional Ashtanga Yoga Primary Series class, and that was the experience that solidified the change in my life. I wasn't athletic or particularly physically fit, and I certainly had no idea what a lineage-based yoga practice was. But I kept practicing because of how I felt when I got off the mat. I also learned that just because you cannot balance in a pose, it does not mean you are not worthy of practicing yoga.

Yoga practice, especially Ashtanga Yoga practice, is anything but easy. We all have met or will most likely meet failure right in our first class. Not only was I not very good at the asanas but I also was not good at failing or falling out of the asanas. Frustration and failure have a nasty habit of sneaking into your mindset, and they have the potential to really ruin your practice if you let them. The reality of staying inspired to practice yoga when you keep failing is exceptionally difficult. Struggle, adversity, and challenge bring dukha in all its shapes and forms. You cannot expect to avoid failure, but what you can do is change the way you think about failure.

Yoga practice is a space where failure is welcome. Failure is the only way you can learn from yoga, because yoga isn't about memorizing or perfecting the poses. It is a personal and spiritual journey that strengthens your mental abilities just as much as—if not more than—your physical form.

What asanas you do (or not) on the mat should not impact the way you feel about your practice. We all need a lesson in being a little bit nicer to ourselves. We cannot judge our success by our asanas; you can succeed at yoga even if you mess up some of the poses! Failing at a pose or two does not mean you are failing at yoga. The real success of the practice comes from the balance you find within yourself when you let go of all the overhanging—and sometimes unrealistic—expectations you put on yourself.

Are you, like me, a perfectionist who is afraid of failure? Fear of failure is a huge inhibition, both on the yoga mat and in your everyday life. This fear can stop you from achieving the things you want most in the world. When you let fear rule your actions, you trap yourself in an endless loop of fear and failure that can be difficult to break. In a success-oriented society like ours, failure can be seen as a threat to our livelihood. Each of us will experience this fear more times than we can count. Rather than pushing us to succeed perfectly, yoga teaches us how to redefine success. When fear of failure and perfectionism kick in, we tend to focus obsessively on goals and results. Yoga instead focuses all our efforts on the process, and the journey opens the mind to be fully present and accept the reality of what exists. Even after more than twenty years of yoga practice, I still have my own doubts when it comes to my abilities as both a student and a teacher. Instead of fighting these feelings, I have learned to acknowledge the doubt, fear, and discomfort and integrate these aspects of myself into both my practice and my life.

Remember—perfection does not exist, and no one will ever achieve it. What you can achieve is self-acceptance and a higher sense of self that is able to accept failure and learn new things because of it. This process of trying-failing-learning is the process-oriented thinking you need to be successful at yoga. Process-oriented thinking in your yoga practice gives you the freedom to not care about whether you achieve the pose and reduces your mind to a focus on the breath and the internal journey.

Truthfully, yoga is hard, process and all. I still find my practice challenging after all these years. Few things worth doing are easy, after all. We all come to yoga practice for different reasons, and there is absolutely nothing wrong with that. Wanting to strengthen your body, open your mind, and improve your health are all great reasons to seek out a yoga studio. Yoga is not a fast and easy shortcut away from suffering. It is a slow and steady journey, and like all journeys, your yoga practice will come with its own deeply personal trials and tribulations. Your job is to unroll the mat and start again.

THE BIRTH OF DISCIPLINE

Building the discipline to practice can be difficult. Some people have a strong reaction to discipline and avoid it. Other people take to discipline almost too easily and wind up with rigidity. To make yoga a lifelong practice, we have to find that perfect balance between discipline and tenderness. We have to learn through trial and error when it is appropriate to apply discipline and when it is appropriate to be gentle. Ashtanga allows you to work with the mind and train it to find this equilibrium within yourself. In the Yoga Sutras, Patanjali presents the concept of *tapas* as a way to build the necessary discipline required to truly devote oneself to yoga. *Tapas* is literally translated into English as "heat" but has a much more nuanced meaning. Tapas comprises the fire, energy, and inspiration that help all students of yoga learn how to break the old unhealthy habits of the past and build new habits of liberation.

Willingly subjecting yourself to heat may sound intense, and tapas is honestly not meant to be easy. In fact, tapas could also be understood as a kind of confrontational process where you meet yourself on your mat. There are many levels of tapas, and the first starts within the physical body. When you feel your muscles burning in a healthy manner (we will talk more about that later), imagine that it is the tapas burning through your body. Tapas becomes more subtle when you start burning through the old states of your personality, and there is often emotional, psychological, or spiritual suffering.

The benefits of tapas start first with the physical body, then move through the energy and space around and within the body, and finally work through the mind and spirit. Tapas will start in *kaya*, the physical body, with all the accompanying sensations that occur. The body is also the realm of automated functions, like digestion and immunological responses, that are governed by the subconscious mind. The body is a reservoir for the subconscious mind. Yoga is about full consciousness, and the physical poses can bring subconscious thoughts to the surface. Once these subconscious thoughts become conscious, the work of purification goes even deeper. When tapas moves to your physical senses, *indriya*, the power of perception, is sharpened. The five senses are more than just a means to experience the external world—they can direct the mind either outward or inward. If the senses remain focused on the external world, happiness will always be dependent on external occurrences. By contrast, once the senses focus on the inner world, happiness and all the accompanying benefits of spiritual practice occur within, independently of what occurs in the external world. To help understand the impact of the focal point of the senses, think of a tornado, spinning violently, destroying everything in its wake. Take this outward energy and focus it inward. Reverse the spin until it slows and eventually comes to a stop. The same power that fueled destruction now illuminates the path of liberation.

Siddhi, which means "actualization," is what occurs after putting in the work of tapas. Every yoga practitioner has had a small taste of the benefits of tapas, even though we may not achieve the full impact of it in this lifetime. The important part is that we put in the work and get on the mat every day to face our egos. The degree to which we are willing to show up for tapas is the degree to which we will work for our own liberation.

The tapas will be strongest during your hardest practice, when you face the biggest and most deeply seeded obstacles, so never let the pain hold you back from showing up on your mat. Whether it is physical or emotional, pain is what leads to this purification and brings up the fire and heat within you. When you feel the burn of suffering, that means your tapas is on fire; my advice is to let it smolder while understanding how to safely work your body and mind.

Successful tapas may or may not result in the attainment of various shapes with the body. It may result in a qualitative change in how you face your own suffering. My goal with this book is to change the whole paradigm of "success." The next time you get on the yoga mat, try thinking about failure and success differently. Learn to see failure in a new light and keep moving forward with your practice. Success is what you get from yoga practice when you learn something about yourself, when there is more sensation in the body, and when you change how you respond to dukha—not necessarily when you do a certain asana in a certain way.

We must remember that tapas is more than just looking for pain and at the same time let go of the common misconception that yoga is supposed to feel good all the time. While the practice often does feel good, seeking pleasure is its own kind of delusion and suffering. Dukha is a dual-edged sword that usually produces either attachment to pleasure or aversion to pain from the same source. Whichever side of the sword you find yourself on, it cuts with the same sharpness. Pleasure can lead to addiction if left unchecked or riddled with attachment. Ashtanga Yoga practice trains us in how to become equanimous with our pain and our pleasure. The only truth is change. Sometimes there is pleasure, sometimes there is pain.

In layman's terms, yoga can be understood as coming from the Sanskrit "yuj" and meaning to unite, add or connect body to spirit/soul. Sanatana dharma can be understood as everlasting or eternal, and dharma as order. Infinite order like yoga, which begins and has no end as it connects you to the infinite within you. Asanas/postures are just work as tools to keep the mechanism of the human body healthy so the ultimate goal can be reached or achieved. Yoga also means a disciplined way of life, and to be a student of yoga isn't easy. Yoga practitioners have to cultivate the discipline to eat on time, sleep on time—no more or less. The yoga path means finding balance in everything, and it does not happen overnight. Yoga takes time, effort, and hard work. This isn't limited to asana practice; it just begins from there and get deeper.

—AJAY TOKAS

Acceptance of the unavoidable and uncontrollable fluctuations between pleasure and pain is the result of many years of practice. That serene and peaceful look on the faces of yogis comes with years of asana practice and meditation that teaches all students how to sit and truly experience all that is without attachment or aversion. Yoga is a path that eventually leads to the transcendence of duality. Running from pain only leads to more misery. Holding on to pleasure ensures its escape.

But yoga is not meant to be only a daily battle. The practice is not designed just to make us push harder or work faster. We are not actively *trying* to generate more experiences of pain. Pain arrives all on its own. Yoga is here to prepare us to overcome the inexorable nature of dukha with grace. We train in how to inhabit uncomfortable spaces without generating more suffering. We learn to recognize how the body and mind react to negative experiences of pain, sadness, hurt, and discomfort. In seeing our own reactions, we gain the perspective necessary to overcome our old patterns.

The truth you may have gleaned by now is that yoga as a spiritual path is not a light, casual endeavor. Many yoga students, including myself, get rather irked by the seemingly incessant presence of dukha in the practice. The teaching tells us that instead of worrying about perfecting the asanas right off the bat, we need to learn to enjoy the process as it develops. It is important, if you are newer to the practice, not to judge yourself against people who have been practicing for a long time. It is equally important for long-term practitioners and teachers to remember to cultivate that beginner's mind.

What matters more than anything else is that we commit to showing up day after day, when it feels good, when it feels bad, when we are inspired, and when we are no longer inspired. Tapas is consistency, dedication, and determination over many years.

Within the practice, there are two opposing forces that must be balanced. One force—*sthira*—is our strength, willpower, and determination. The second, *sukha*, is the ease and flow of the practice, the force that represents happiness and comfort. Truly embodying both these aspects seems like a contradiction, yet that is exactly what is required. We must learn how to be determined yet maintain a comfortable ease and flow in our yoga practice. We cannot be too strict with ourselves, but we also cannot be so lenient that we don't complete a single pose. Finding the balance in our yoga practice is the true success we should be working toward.

Calming the mind is at the root of our yoga practice. The route to tranquility lies not in the annihilation of every source of irritation outside ourselves but in containing the opposing forces of pleasure and pain within. Ashtanga Yoga uses the trinity of breath, body, and mind working together as tools that allow us to build the foundation of a calm and peaceful state of mind. Sooner or later, after much practice, it will happen for every practitioner. There is joy within every yogic experience we have along the journey, whether we face stormy or serene sailing. We can learn how to maintain two seemingly contradictory experiences within ourselves, and we can hold that tension within our minds. Tapas might be seen as the dynamic balance of the living paradox within us, and the realization of tapas could be seen as spiritual intelligence.

HACK YOUR BRAIN WITH YOGA

Yoga was traditionally referred to as a science of liberation. There are elements of yoga that can be studied and verified by rational, scientific means. There are also mystical elements that can only be experienced directly. Retraining our brains and bodies sits at the juncture between the scientific and the mystical. There are measurable results that can occur from yoga practice, and there are inexplicable changes that happen when we practice. What is unarguable is that we have the power to train both the body and mind, and that power resides definitively within ourselves.

To visualize this, think of the Native American parable of the two wolves. As the story goes, two wolves live in each of us—the wolf of hate powered by anger, sorrow, jealousy, and greed; and the wolf of love powered by compassion, peace, love, and forgiveness. These two wolves are in direct competition with one another. Which one survives is up to us. The wolf that lives is the one we feed. Each breath is a choice, just as each action is a choice. When we breathe and act unconsciously, we often feed the destructive wolf. When we breathe and act with awareness, we have a chance to feed the sanguine wolf. The evidence of a successful yoga practice shows up when we become kinder and more empathetic toward ourselves and others.

It would be a mistake to think of the two wolves as enemies. When we see the destructive wolf arising, we cannot wage a war against that being. Instead, we are tasked with radically accepting the wolf as it is and simultaneously growing our relationship with the sanguine wolf. While much of yogic philosophy focuses on suffering and pain, there is an equal amount of work to be done in nurturing the systems of connection, empathy, and compassion. The wolf of love is the state of calm and connection we all feel in our practice. The physical poses of yoga are designed to develop our empathy and our kindness, and it behooves us to remember this as we practice.

The spiritual journey of yoga uses the tool of asana to train the mind and build new patterns of thinking. The more you practice yoga, the stronger your mind becomes. With increased power comes increased responsibility. With each asana, you build a concentrated mind that has the potential to develop new, more compassionate patterns. With practice, you can learn to reconceptualize the way you think about yourself, your yoga practice, and your whole world. With a mind unfettered from the chains of attachment and aversion, you can see clearly and develop your natural capacity for empathy. The lesson of the two wolves boils down to discerning that we have the power to change the way we think.

While it might sound a bit odd, I genuinely believe we can learn to use yoga as a kind of life hack. Think about all your accumulated thoughts, patterns, emotions, and behaviors as a kind of software installed in the hardware of the body and mind. This software runs the programming of your life, and it has largely been installed unconsciously. To bring consciousness into every thought, emotion, and behavior, the mind needs to be hacked. If you have ever heard of jailbreaking a phone, then perhaps you can think of yoga as the tool that allows you to break into the hardware of the mind and install a new program. Yoga practice can open you up to a new life of infinite growth and inner peace by teaching your brain (and your body) new ways of thinking. Your tendencies toward self-hatred and negative thinking are not permanent states of being. The operating system of your brain can be updated, and you can become a conscious creator of the thoughts you think and the emotions you feel.

In ancient times, yoga practitioners in India developed the practice to understand the operating system of the human mind—they referred to the methodology of yoga as spiritual science. The word *science* is defined in English as a systematic study of the world through observation and experimentation. Instead of studying the world outside of themselves, ancient yogis studied the world within themselves. If we apply their methodology in our contemporary world, we might even call yoga a kind of technology. Yoga has always been referred to as a science of self-realization to distinguish it amongst the many branches of spiritual philosophies within India's historic past. Thinking of the body as hardware, our patterned thinking as software, our accumulated paradigm as the operating system, and the practice of yoga as a hack to the system mainframe, we can also think of language as a kind of code base. Language is more than words. Much of our communication happens with our bodies, and almost all of our body language is subconscious. The body's language is intricately connected with the power of the subconscious mind. In spoken words, the conscious mind rules, but when your mind is silent, the body still speaks with candor.

In the Ashtanga Yoga method, silence and quiet form the passage to the subconscious mind. If you practice alone at home or join a traditional Mysore-style class, one of the things you will notice first is how little is said. The absence of noise creates an atmosphere of introspection that lets you step into and through your body with each asana. If yoga is going to hack the system, the hacker needs access to the deepest layers of programming that exist within the body and subconscious mind. Communicating with your body is key to using yoga as a life hack. One of the reasons teachers recommend practicing yoga first thing in the morning is because it is easier to penetrate beyond the surface layer of the mind before the hustle and bustle of the day kicks in.

Learning to speak the language of the body is like learning to write code. Instead of all the symbols of code base, the body speaks through sensations. Feeling every cell and fiber of the body is the first step to updating your subconscious mind and the way you think about yourself and the world around you. The unfelt body is unconscious, unloved, and asleep. While not every asana feels good, every asana succeeds when you are left with more sensation. Each sensation that arises in the body can be met with neutrality instead of reactivity. The old pattern of the mind falsely assumes that the source of permanent happiness exists when external circumstances are pleasurable. The new pattern of the mind sees pleasure and pain as temporary experiences that are constantly in flux. This departure from cycles of suffering is as radical as jailbreaking your phone.

The thinking mind operates in words, but your body is communicating in a space that is not words. When you try a new pose, you access a new body language and body intelligence. It doesn't matter whether you ever perform that asana in a particular aesthetic shape. It matters that you leave the pose with increased body sensations and an equanimous mind.

THE KNOWLEDGE RIDDLE

Identification with the mind and body is a source of suffering according to traditional yoga philosophy. Whether we identify with our thoughts or our bodies, neither of them are the truth of who we are. Both the body and the mind are in a constant state of flux. Life is more than this material structure. Detaching our self-identity from our bodies, thoughts, and emotions subverts the entire basis of identity. Almost like an operation of the mind, the shift must be performed with surgical precision. The goal of yoga practice is to do just that—shift the focal point of your identification and then allow you to experience for yourself what exists beyond mind and matter.

You are not your body. You are not your thoughts. You are not your emotions. You experience all these things. You have access to the body as an avatar on earth. If you cling to these material manifestations, you limit your sense of self and further entrench yourself within the cycles of suffering. The ego glorifies itself by holding on desperately to specific thoughts, emotions, and bodily sensations. Furthering the desires of the ego is antithetical to the work of yoga. When you step on the mat and begin your practice, you make a statement that you are ready to wake up to the truth of who you really are. The fact that you are reading this book means that a very deep place within you is already working for your own liberation. This is no mundane feat, so take a moment to validate your own efforts so far.

Understating the three types of knowledge presented by Patanjali's sutras will help you navigate the more subtle aspects of the inner work of yoga:

- **ANUMANA**, or intellectual knowledge, is what you can think about and reach with a seemingly logical conclusion.

- **AGAMA**, or devotional knowledge, is the knowledge you don't understand but take to be true because you trust the source.

- **PRAMANA**, or experiential knowledge, is knowledge born from direct experience, and it happens when you know something to be true because you have experienced it yourself.

Ideally, these types of knowledge all line up and we reach a transcendent sense of self-knowledge. But too often we reach incorrect logical conclusions or devote ourselves to the wrong sources of information. At some point in history all available knowledge indicated that the earth was flat. Logic, devotional knowledge, and direct experience all pointed to this erroneous conclusion. We unfortunately follow similarly erroneous paths in our daily lives without realizing it—our false knowledge then often exacerbates our misconception of ourselves.

We have all come to an incorrect logical conclusion at some point in our lives. It is humbling to realize that you can use logic and still reach a wrong conclusion that looks and feels correct. Even if we confirm our conclusions with another source, that source may engage in the same inaccurate evaluations. We thus end up devoting ourselves to a misconception. In our contemporary age of alternative facts and fake news, it's easy to get duped by sources that appear to be trustworthy. There are many stories of people who follow a fake news story only to feel utterly disillusioned when the actual truth is revealed. It may feel natural to give your trust to an authority figure you idolize and lose your sense of right and wrong. When I was first starting yoga, I believed a teacher who said that they only ate apples. They presented me with a lot of information that appeared plausible regarding a single-source food diet. I tried and failed to eat only apples and felt awful about my failure. But one day I discovered that my teacher was supplementing their diet with all sorts of things, including Oreo cookies! I felt simultaneously relieved and embarrassed. What we choose to believe is powerful. Choice is the liberating factor that comes with its own burdens.

Reconceptualizing the basis of knowledge is not an easy shift in thought process. In yoga the purpose of thinking critically about epistemology is not simply intellectual gymnastics. Instead, yoga seeks to reveal the timeless truth of beingness. It is qualitatively more than just turning around to get a new perspective. The challenge lies in breaking the habits of the mind to think beyond the physical and the mental. Shifting this thought process is a goal of yoga practice. Only when we realize that we are not our thoughts, emotions, or bodies do we have the power to truly understand what the mind and body actually are. Only when we understand that the source of suffering is not outside but within us, then we finally have the power to work with our pain. What we accept as reality makes a very big impact on how we feel day-to-day. If we are unable to come to an estimation of what is true ourselves, then our minds so easily accept the unconscious biases that have been programmed into society that we unwittingly become copies of the world we live in.

The search for knowledge is the search for truth and liberation—it is the essence of yoga. *Satya* is a Sanskrit word that means "true essence" or "truthfulness." The goal of yoga is to cultivate satya, and I would like to flush out this concept a bit.

Satya is not only objective truth; it also includes the ethical concept of the value of truthfulness. Satya is considered a virtue of yoga practice, and it guides us on our own quest for truth. More importantly, satya is the opposite of falsehood and delusion, and it helps govern the very operation of our universe.

The yoga quest seeks the answers to some of the deepest questions of life. The goal of yoga is to cultivate true knowingness about ourselves and the whole world. Satya exists in our individual actions and thoughts, and it can influence the way we interact with one another. By practicing yoga, we can move on from our individual biased truths and into the universal truths of this reality. Universal truths—like the sun rises in the east and sets in the west—are infallible. On the other hand, our individual truths are shaped by our experiences and are often fungible and misguided. What we take to be truths are often based on value judgments and opinions. We make most of these judgments subconsciously, which can give people the power to take advantage of our relative truths. Yoga aims to find you a path out of this relative truth through the practice of satya.

Seeing clearly is harder than we think. So often what we think is true is in fact just our opinion, and our opinion is so often skewed by our past experiences. Instead of seeing clearly, we see from behind our own fog. Then we take actions based on faulty assumptions, and big surprise, our actions lead to more suffering and confusion. Without spiritual practice, we remain caught in cycles of delusion that worsen and intensify over time. Spiritual practice aims to clear the mind so we can finally make evaluations based on the actual experience of reality. Instead of seeing things based on our opinions, judgments, and past, we see things as they truly are. Only when we are free from the baggage of our patterns can we hope to take actions that will lead to less suffering, more peace, and ultimately liberation.

Are we perfect? Absolutely not. We stumble and fall and make mistakes. But the key is that spiritual practice is just that—practice.

SEEKING: CONSCIOUSLY OR UNCONSCIOUSLY

The secret to yoga practice is how we use the asanas. These poses we twist our bodies into are not just for our physical health and strength. Yoga practice has the power to lead us on a path of liberation from the mind *and* body. While our subconscious minds are made up of the habitual reactions of our thoughts, bodies, and emotions, yoga can tap into and disrupt even the most negative cycles of thinking.

How? Consider this: rather than thinking of the brain and mind as synonymous, consider the theory that the mind is actually capable of creating reality based on our perception. This perception includes our innate physical reactions to certain stimuli, such as pain or pleasure. For example, when something is uncomfortable, our reaction is to run away or otherwise remove ourselves from the painful situation. But if you practice yoga, you are training yourself to remain neutral in the face of discomfort.

The discomfort we experience on the yoga mat is there to teach us how to recognize our response to these bodily sensations. Yoga teaches us that it is not the pain that defines us. Instead, the way we react to pain is what will determine the direction of our lives. Learning how *not* to react is one of the most important lessons you will learn on the yoga mat. Mastering your response to pain will give you the ability to change the way you think, and that is the first step toward changing your habits and becoming the best possible version of yourself. Every single person that interacts with the discipline of yoga is, in some ways, a spiritual seeker. The whole premise of yoga is predicated on the notion that you need a personal practice as a forum for you to experience some of these esoteric, more mystical truths.

Every one of us must ask ourselves (sometimes more than once): *What is yoga?* Your spiritual quest is just that—a journey. It is always important to learn the historical context of yoga and apply the methodology of yoga to your practice so you understand it's not just a lot of stretching and lifting.

Prakriti and *purusha* are the dichotomy at the center of Patanjali's teachings. Prakriti—the phenomenal world—is our material world, the ephemeral where the only constant is change. On the flip side is purusha—the noumenal world—which is the singularity that exists independently of our sense and perception; it is that oneness we seek within ourselves and with our universe. According to Patanjali, both prakriti and purusha are within us all. The seed of suffering begins with the fundamental ignorance about what is prakriti and what is purusha. Or, to put it more plainly, we suffer because we have forgotten who we really are. The oneness within us now identifies itself as our bodies or our thoughts. When purusha thinks it is prakriti, everything gets skewed and misunderstood. Yoga practice aims to give each practitioner the light of knowledge and discrimination, or the ability to delineate between what is true and untrue. Yoga is a quest for the liberating light within. Without this philosophical framework, yoga can be misunderstood as just a lot of body bending or, worse, a way for us to ignore reality. Yoga teaches us that we are not helpless victims of our life experiences. We are so much more than the names and forms we so often identify with.

One of my biggest lessons on the yoga mat was (and sometimes still is) the acceptance of the inevitable shifts between pleasure and pain. More than that, it's being able to sit in the reality of change with a relaxed and nonjudgmental attitude. We have the power to break our subconscious thinking patterns if we learn to accept the ups and downs in the practice. The spiritual journey is made up of struggles. Yoga is a practice, not a performance. It is an opportunity to learn.

2

Being Part of Something Greater

YOGA IS PHYSICAL PRACTICE with a spiritual intent. The real tools of the spiritual path let you go into the ecstatic highs and the anguish-filled lows with the understanding that nothing is permanent.

RELEARNING THE LANGUAGE OF THE BODY

If we feel uncomfortable in our skin, there is no escape from that. There will be no peace anywhere we go. Asana practice helps us bring the mind fully into the body. Along the way we will have to make peace with all the places where we feel uncomfortable in our bodies.

We all come to the yoga mat for many different reasons. We crave a healthier lifestyle, or we believe we're ready to take on the spiritual journey of yoga practice. Regardless of where we come from, the yoga journey will lead us all into meeting our bodies, sometimes for the first time.

Meeting your body—more importantly, loving your body and being comfortable in your own skin—is one of the biggest blessings that comes from yoga practice. We spend so much time in our minds and outside our physical forms that we have forgotten how to actually be inside our bodies. Yoga is a tool that can reacquaint you with yourself and teach you how to be comfortable in your body. There is a sense of ease that comes from being at home in your own skin. You cannot run and hide from yourself, and you cannot escape the body as long as you remain on earth, even though we all may have tried at some point. To find peace, we have to be at peace within our bodies and within ourselves.

Before I started practicing yoga, I had no prior physical training. In some sense I was a foreigner within my own body. I did not speak the language of the body, and I did not know how the body worked. There were sensations, feelings, and movements that all occurred subconsciously. Worse still, if I had any relationship with my body, it was one of antagonism. Instead of feeling and accepting my body, all I wanted to do was change it so that it fit into a particular mold. Even when I started yoga, I was still at a kind of war with my body. Since I could not do many of the poses and the whole practice was so difficult, I blamed my body, got frustrated with my size and shape, and wished I had trained in some physical discipline when I was a child. It took years of practice before I could sign a peace treaty between my ego and my body. Since I know how damaging it can be to live in turmoil, my sincere wish for every student of yoga is that they find the path to peace. The more we are at peace with ourselves, the more we will be at peace with one another. Each of us needs to find out what it means to be at home in our own skin. It is not an instantaneous shift. It is a process that unfolds over years of practice, much like gaining fluency in a new language.

The body does not speak with grammar or logic in the same way that the mind does. The body will speak through sensation and feeling. The body's voice is more subtle. More importantly, the body's voice is friendly. No matter how much conflict there has been between the mind and the body, the body has never stopped trying to do its best for you. Whenever there is disease and pain, the body tries its best to heal. Whatever fuel it is given, it uses to the best of its ability. In fact, our bodies have been speaking to us all since we were born, but we have forgotten this ancient language. Coming to the yoga mat can help us remember or relearn how to listen to the intelligence of the body. The biggest mistake so many yoga students make is failing to realize that they have the inner potential to love themselves and be comfortable in their own skin. We can unlearn stories of hate and judgment. Each time you get on the mat, change the paradigm of worthiness through achievement by truly listening and tuning in to your body's language. Then, yoga will take you on a journey to become best friends with your body.

DECONSTRUCTING AND RECONSTRUCTING

By now it should be abundantly clear that yoga is not just a physical practice. Our value, skill, and worth is not only limited to our physical frame. We are practicing yoga to be a part of something greater than ourselves. To get to this pivotal point of awareness, it might be useful to deconstruct some of the hierarchical language that is sometimes heard in the yoga classroom. Whether teacher or student, we all hear various cues that call out alignment points and directions for yoga poses. If the language we use as teachers or hear as students is hierarchical in nature, there may be unintended stress and harm. To start off, you may have noticed that I have used the word *adaptation* rather than *modification* to refer to the various ways that a pose can be made accessible to different yoga practitioners. While it may seem like a small semantic difference, to me it means a lot. When we modify something, there is an implicit assumption that a correct and more worthy whole exists out there somewhere. It sets an unspoken standard of

There is much intelligence behind the Ashtanga curriculum, but when we hold the curriculum too rigidly, the intelligence dries up. Honoring that intelligence means allowing our practices to change and evolve in whatever way necessary, so the creative force can move openly through our bodies. This is the future of Ashtanga, the direction in which we, as long-term practitioners of Ashtanga, must evolve—becoming more supple, more generous, more forgiving in our approach, and above all, more immediately receptive to the wild intelligence of the body.

—TY LANDRUM

perfection that only a privileged few may one day attain. Similarly, when we refer to the "full expression" of a pose being only one way, we relegate all others to being seen as less-than. But adapting something is qualitatively different. Instead of the student who needs to change, it is the pose itself that needs to change to better serve the student. The power dynamic is flipped, and the unattainable standard gets dethroned. Implicit subconscious judgments are often expressed in language. We are not often aware of the framework that forms the linguistic basis of speech. When we suggest that "stiff" or "weak" people do one thing while "flexible" or "strong" people do another, we create divisions and spark jealousy. When we value one expression of a pose over another, we foster an attitude of competition. While it may seem harmless, this kind of qualifying language inspires the idea that some poses are more important than others or, worse, that some yogis aren't working as hard as others.

You cannot tell how hard someone is working on the yoga mat just by looking at them, and it is the teacher's job to create a space where everyone can practice yoga comfortably and safely. If you are a teacher, seek out trainings that provide guidance in how to use more inclusive words in the classroom. Modern language has come a long way, but there are still many steps to take on this path. Numerous common expressions and cues often exclude gender nonconforming people. Greeting others, whether as teacher or student, with "Hey, guys," may not be as friendly as we think it is. Instead, just "Hey," or "Hey, friends," gives space for everyone to be seen. If you are a student, seek out a teacher whose conscious use of language makes you feel safe and who gives you the space to explore the options that work best for you. The correct version of a pose is the one that works for you today.

The false equivalence of physical aptitude with spiritual depth stems from a misinterpretation and misunderstanding of the ancient teachings of yoga. To overcome this, we have to dive deeply into the hidden biases within ourselves. We are not in the yoga room to show off or "outpose" anyone else; we are here to learn, to practice, and to become better human beings so we can bring the goodness needed to make a positive change in this world.

SPIRITUAL BYPASSING

As people who are active in the world—as we are even on this yogic journey—we are still contributing to the greater society. As yogis, it is our job to look at how we can make a difference. Yet even within the spiritual community there are pitfalls that contort the teachings. Along these lines, *spiritual bypassing* is an important term for every teacher and student of yoga. Understanding this concept is integral to your journey as it may be what's holding you back from your spiritual growth through yoga.

Spiritual bypassing was originally introduced by John Welwood in the 1980s to describe the process that happens when certain concepts of the spiritual path are co-opted and used for avoidance, repression, and other negative mechanisms. All the concepts we learn about in yoga—patience, positivity, acceptance, enlightenment—can be hijacked by our old tendencies without us even realizing it.

One of the most common expressions that illustrates a spiritual bypass is when people use the phrase "love and light" as a means to disregard negative feedback or other uncomfortable situations. If you ever find yourself thinking negative thoughts and feeling guilty about it, you are experiencing a spiritual bypass. If you ever think that yogis should not be angry, sad, anxious, or otherwise imperfect, you are experiencing a spiritual bypass. In this paradigm the shadow self is banished and judged. While it can be difficult to sit and acknowledge the pain of the shadow side of ourselves, rejecting any portion of ourselves ignites another cycle of suffering. In moments of insecurity, frustration, or anger, the body and mind get flooded and overloaded. In that moment, the idea that "everything is fine" and we just need to "breathe" can feel disingenuous or even offensive. We cannot pretend that problems do not exist, but we can take control of the way we feel about the problems.

The spiritual tools of yoga are meant to give you the confidence to go into the deepest darkness of your shadow self with the understanding that nothing is permanent. There is real harm in the world. Ignoring it or pretending it does not exist is not a solution. There is real suffering—physical, mental, environmental, economic, and more. When an idea that you "should" be happy collides with the harsh reality of your experience, the real work of yoga can help you find the way to a stable foundation. But the spiritual bypass is just an escape, a way to mask discomfort with the shadow. At best, it is an ill-fitting Band-Aid that just does not fit over the wound of suffering. At worst, it aggravates the injury. Detachment does not mean nothing matters. In fact, the opposite is true: everything matters, and our task is to feel and be present to everything with calm, clear minds and open hearts.

A spiritual bypass is not always immediately evident. The path to enlightenment contains many byways where we can potentially veer off course. All we can do is our best. With the help of our teachers and our community, we can commit ourselves to the total journey of yoga.

UNPACKING PRIVILEGE

Any discussion of accessibility in Ashtanga Yoga has to include the question of who is dominant in the yoga space and why. Accessibility means deconstructing the paradigm of privilege that assumes that only a certain subset of society should have access to yoga practice. Privilege includes economic,

Accessibility is a matter of power. Who has access and who doesn't. When it comes to cultural traditions, who has the power to represent, "gate keep," and grant access and who has the power to gain access. Imagining the future of Ashtanga Yoga or proposing reforms to the tradition, we would do well to consider the complex power dynamics that led to the global popularity of Ashtanga Yoga.

—GREG NARDI

racial, social, gender, and physical advantages that exist in an insidious state of the status quo. It is not enough to say that yoga is for everyone. We must actively change the paradigm so yoga can truly be for all.

There is an intersection of yoga practice and social justice that manifests in the call to work for accessibility. Challenging the dominant image of who a yoga practitioner is requires questioning the mainstream narrative of wellness and pioneering a new type of yoga space.

In many yoga classes, there are often few people of color, neurodivergent people, disabled students, or queer folx. Lack of representation causes real harm. Cultures that are based on inequity are built on harm and cause trauma. Within this context, we must acknowledge that historically yoga has not been accessible to everyone.

This is not a question of whether yoga students and teachers are good people or not. There is a difference between being passively good as opposed to being actively engaged in the spiritual practice of deconstruction and evolution.

We all can learn to recognize the roles we play in different situations. Having power and privilege colors our experiences, and it is important to ask ourselves, "Where do I experience privilege?" both on and off the yoga mat. This exercise is not meant to generate shame but to develop a sense of awareness so we can use our perspective to create change. This quest is really the essence of yogic values translated into everyday life. We are in the world, we are embodied, and our yoga practice should touch all parts of our lives. Yoga is not something we are doing externally. It is a practice we are trying to embody in daily life. We have to have humility in our practice, and we have to have humility as yoga teachers and students.

Over the past twenty years, we have seen the yoga world morph and evolve, yet there is always more work to do. It has taken us this long to recognize the need to support and uplift the totality of voices in our yoga community. So many people start yoga because it seems like an interesting workout that just so happens to be sprinkled with spiritual teachings. It often is not until students hear the Yoga Sutras for the first time that they recognize the true spiritual power of the yoga journey or acknowledge the practice's origin culture.

I believe in accessible yoga classes that welcome people from every racial, religious, gender, physical, and socioeconomic demographic to practice the asanas and explore their own yoga journeys. Yoga class is ideally a place where people can come to practice, relax, and enjoy themselves. For many people, this is rarely the case.

yuvo vṛddho|ativṛddho vā vyādhito durbalo|api vā |
abhyāsātsiddhimāpnoti sarva-yogheshvatandritah ||1. 67

Whether young, old or too old, sick or lean, one who discards laziness and gets success if he practices Yoga.

—*Hatha Yoga Pradipika*

Unlike the *Hatha Yoga Pradipika* quotation, we rarely see elderly, disabled, or bigger-bodied students practicing yoga. Think about it—when you do a Google search for "yoga," there are mostly images of white, able-bodied, young, thin, neurotypical women. Think about what kind of message this sends to yoga students and also how it affects their and your own yoga journey. If you do not see yourself in the yoga community, then it will be hard to truly feel like you are a part of that community.

Ashtanga Yoga in particular does not have a reputation for being accessible, and I have spent the last few years of teaching trying to change this. Yoga teachers have to learn how to teach classes that welcome people of all ages, body types, skin colors, and genders. This experience is something many teachers lack, and we need better training to create accessibility in yoga. Students can pioneer creating spaces that support their communities in practice groups, yoga clubs, and online groups.

If yoga practice is only a place for high ponytails, skinny waists, and light skin, then this leaves very little room for diversity. It should be said that there is no problem per se with high ponytails, skinny waists, or light skin. It is only an issue if that's all there is. There are many ways in which the media perpetuates these images and ultimately deters many people from ever stepping foot in a studio. People who look different often get treated differently. According to traditional yoga philosophy, all beings have the innate potential for liberation and enlightenment. All beings are equally worthy on a spiritual level. It is up to yoga teachers and students to work toward a yoga community where we truly embody the lofty principles of our philosophy.

Ashtanga Yoga, like most yoga practices popularly taught and practiced around the world today, is a Brahmanical tradition. Since I started my yoga journey, I have oscillated between the dilemma of being from a marginalized community whose separation was written (or rather omitted because the untouchables weren't worthy of a mention) into the sacred scriptures of yoga and the benefit that this practice has on me. Unlike many Western students, I could not take an absolutist view of the yogic scriptures. Instead, my identity as coming from outside the power structure allowed me to apply a more rational and less devotional paradigm to the teachings. As students of yoga committed to the path of ahimsa, readers, practitioners, and seekers, this is also what we need to realize—that some of the scriptures being referred to us for our spiritual journey through classical yoga philosophy are also works of fiction. What the practitioners must also be aware of and grow sensitive toward are the repercussions of these scriptures in Indian society.

—MEETALI MESHRAM

3

Fostering Growth

THE ROLE OF YOGA—and our responsibility as yogis—is to evolve. Yoga is a path of action. Justice is more than just love, light, hopes, and prayers. When we update the framework of our thinking and embody the practice of yoga in our lives, the natural next step is to codify this change in our deeds. This book is meant to inspire you and equip you with the knowledge you may need to move forward with these changes. The true philosophy and spirituality of yoga unlocks the limitless potential for fostering growth.

AHIMSA 2.0

Ahimsa is a core yogic principle introduced by Patanjali in the Yoga Sutras as the first of the moral and ethical precepts that yoga aspirants are advised to follow. *Ahimsa* means "nonviolence," but it is much more than merely not committing harm. When an *a* is placed in front of a word in Sanskrit, that turns the word into its opposite. *Himsa* is the Sanskrit word for "violence," so ahimsa is not only nonviolence but the opposite of violence. Perhaps this means that if harm is being done to any of our fellow human beings, then as yogis it is our responsibility to be of service and do what we can to correct the course. Maybe ahimsa has the magic of a personal revolution if we follow the principle of nonviolence toward all living beings to its soteriological end. When we carve out a path of nonviolence in a world filled with violence, we diverge from the status quo in significant ways. Our actions could potentially disrupt the cycle of tacit acceptance that perpetuates violence. At the very least, we will do no harm. At the best, we will do some good.

Maybe ahimsa is kindness, awareness, consideration, and grace. Maybe ahimsa is justice and reconciliation. Maybe ahimsa is peaceful meditation that rights the wrongs of the past. Maybe ahimsa is change for the better.

Yoga practice is designed to break the cycle of suffering. Discrimination is key when applying ahimsa to action. Wrong but well-intentioned actions can still cause harm. The lowest bat for ahimsa means that actions taken will not lead to more suffering. While we may be inspired to immediately apply this teaching to the world, yoga practice always advises us to start with ourselves. Only when we can sit with our own anger, fear, or hatred can we find the path out of it. Until we can resolve the conflict within, we may be less than adequate at resolving the conflict outside ourselves. But that doesn't mean we shouldn't try.

No singular experience should define the entire yoga community. There are unconscious biases built into the business standards of the yoga world that, quite frankly, do not create a safe space for all yogis to learn or even teach their practice. More than that, these biases greatly limit the opportunities yoga students and teachers have to interact with diversity.

It is the responsibility of yoga teachers and studio owners to be present with difficult conversations. As leaders, we need to be open to receiving feedback and constructive criticism. As students, we need to courageously share what our experience is like coming into the yoga space.

There are different ways that yoga teachers can engage with their students and ask these kinds of questions—not only to make sure they and their yoga practice are doing well but also to see where we, as teachers, can create more space and opportunities for all students to get the most from our yoga community. There are ways that yoga students can find the strength to speak to their teachers and communities about what's missing. Some people are afraid to speak up because they do not want to rock the boat, stick out, or ruin the "fun" for everyone else. However, acknowledging places of harm that have occurred within the community of spiritual practitioners allows healing to begin. The strength to lift up into a handstand in yoga is meaningless if we do not also have the strength to show up for challenging community work. Normalizing the process around privilege makes it possible to take one more step toward equity. Silence and shutting down discussion of the issue merely perpetuates the harm that has taken place.

It's not easy to look inward at yourself and start unpacking unconscious prejudice. Maybe a first step in bringing a new level of ahimsa into our yoga communities begins with acknowledging the harm that has been done. We all want to make positive changes, and no one likes admitting that they have caused someone else pain. Being honest about the status quo is perhaps the best foundation for change and growth. We can still embrace ahimsa while taking actions that benefit the whole yoga community and bring the systemic issues we struggle with to the surface.

There is no lasting change without behavioral change on a personal level. I do not claim to be an expert on race relations or sociological theories, but I do have more than twenty years of experience on this spiritual yoga journey. As yoga practitioners, you and I have the power and

If we're going to talk about liberation, we must talk about oppression.
If we're going to access healing,
then we must invite in our wound-
ing. If we're going to clear out in
the light, then we must trust in the
fertile darkness. If we are going to
live for life, then we must die to
death. All too often, our habituation
to an ableist world means that we're
situated in a paradigm that pro-
poses health and wellness to mean
nondisabled. We, the "normal," the
"neurotypical," and nondisabled,
center ourselves in the conversation
around how to "make space" for
neurodivergent and disabled people
in the already existing structures
and paradigms that benefit us.
Disability justice dreams of a future
that is disabled.

—WAMBUI NJUGUNA-RÄISÄNEN

the responsibility to inspire change in our community and to change
ourselves. Reflecting on the need for change is important. Too often the
instinct is to react defensively rather than to listen and reflect. Be strong
enough to listen, especially when it hurts. The rumbles of awakening are
not always smooth and easy. These conversations are uncomfortable,
but discomfort does not equal a lack of safety. Thinking that all the other
obstacles will eventually just go away on their own is delusional. It's a little
like pretending that a heart attack will just resolve itself and not seeking
treatment. Willful ignorance can sometimes be at least as harmful as intentional harm and often harder to identify.

When we stay quiet about our suffering, we let fear and hatred win.
When we speak out about the harm we have experienced or caused, we
align ourselves with consciousness and liberation. As long as unconscious
patterns of harm remain, we will have more work to do in order to embody
justice and peace. And as long as good people continue to turn away from
injustice, lasting peace will never be our reality. But there is great power at
the intersection of spiritual practice and social justice. We have the power
to inspire change in our community, because yoga philosophy is actually
quite radical. We aren't just sending light and love with each pose. In yoga,
love is an action verb, and there are actions we can take as yogis to make
sure those seeds of suffering don't fructify.

CHANGE MAKERS

There are expedient things we can do personally to shift the narrative
today. A dynamic tension accelerates the need to deconstruct the systems
that live in each and every one of us. We are invited to view systems of
oppression as blocking our own personal liberation with the understanding that the oppression of one is the oppression of all.

It is not an either/or equation; the journey is both/and. We can simultaneously question the structures of dominant ideologies and dedicate
ourselves to personal contemplative practice. We can choose to show up
both for ourselves and for the world, working hand in hand, step-by-step
on both fronts.

We are all somewhere and somehow participating in some form of
oppression, myself included. This is hard news to accept, especially for
people who do not feel privileged in any way. Sometimes oppression
appears as internalized racism or disconnection from others' ancestry
instead of overt discrimination or harmful acts. Some practitioners think
the conversation around inequality does not belong in yoga. They say we
should just breathe and stretch and try to feel good. This is the essence
of a spiritual bypass. Behavioral patterns called *samskaras* are expressed
culturally, politically, and economically within our bodies and our society. The world in which we live is not separate from our spiritual practice.
There is a disproportionate representation of privilege in yoga spaces, and

if we want that to change, we have to take action. Marginalized people are often set up to fail in structural oppression. People in the yoga community sometimes miss this. There is a grain of individualistic liberalism that views spirituality in a vacuum, as a personal journey removed from society. Most contemporary yoga practitioners do not realize that there are two paths to take—one that leads back into society and one that leads away from society. The renunciant moves away from society and rejects name, place, and all attachment to the world. Few modern yoga students in the West follow this path. Instead, most Westerners, myself included, are on the path of integration with society and, as such, are charged with doing all they can to make both themselves and the world a better place.

If spiritual practice is only an individual path of enlightenment, then that may miss the point. If we are on the path of liberation and living in the world, then perhaps our spirituality can also include a collective and social sense of awareness. No matter how alone we feel, this is not an entirely solitary journey. Yoga can be both an intensely personal practice and a space of collective healing. By including both the personal and the global, we challenge the dominant ideology with our spiritual practice. The dominant ideology is the water in which we swim, the air we breathe. The dominant ideology is the most powerful samskara that we can challenge, question, and dismantle. The limits defined by the status quo are learned behaviors that force limitless human beings into limited versions of their whole selves.

We have reached a point as a society where passive conversations and empty promises are no longer acceptable. There are steps we can take as yoga teachers, studio owners, students, and human beings to bring about positive change. Unfortunately, when you don't see people who look like you in your yoga classes, it's hard to find the kind of support you need. It can be even harder to approach a yoga teacher or come back to a second class when you don't see yourself in the community.

So many of us practice yoga to heal. We practice yoga to make ourselves stronger—physically, mentally, and spiritually. I first came to the yoga mat in search of something that would make me a *better* person. So it can be very hard for a yoga student to process the all-too-true reality that the yoga community is not the perfect place we hoped it would be.

There is still a lack of diversity in the yoga community, yet many yoga students and teachers have a hard time recognizing this issue. There is a kind of cognitive dissonance between the practice and the world off the mat. Change won't happen overnight, but when you actually take time to enact change in your own way of thinking and living, you will quickly see how those positive changes influence the world around you. A cross-section of a balanced yoga room would ideally reflect the broader society, spanning different ages, shapes, sizes, skin colors, genders, and religions.

Some people might think that we have to throw out the foundation of the status quo to build something new. Instead, perhaps by questioning

Avoiding our pain is a shared human reaction. Yet we can't just dull out the hard stuff and still keep the good stuff. We can't have it both ways. When we numb our pain, we also desensitize our potential to experience everything positive we seek, like happiness, belonging, and connection. Working through what comes up in our yoga practice helps connect us back to ourselves and to each other. As someone in recovery, teaching yoga has been an avenue for me to contribute to society and make a meaningful impact. No one else can do the work for you. You have to show up. But that doesn't mean you're alone. I've seen firsthand that there's a lot of strength in community. When we can talk about the hard things openly, together we have the opportunity to rewrite society's perception of the heavy burdens we carry, like our pain, addiction, mental health issues, and trauma. This shift in how we see things can happen on a bigger scale too. The Ashtanga practice and the benefits it cultivates hold the potential to create profound and lasting change. We can foster a culture of collective well-being and spiritual growth. Our community can help make healing accessible to all. Together we can break through the limiting and isolating barriers of addiction to inspire hope and foster a sense of unity that transcends individual struggles.

—TAYLOR HUNT

the assumptions of the current system, we can update the model without totally eviscerating it. Just like the debris and detritus of the forest floor creates the fertile ground for the next iteration of the forest, we can build on the remnants of the past. Yoga is going to be different for everyone, but yoga *is* for everyone. No matter who you are or where you are on your spiritual path, yoga can bring you the balance you need.

The real work of social awakening goes well beyond the yoga mat. For many people, their first yoga class was a game changer. It altered their whole perspective because they realized they weren't as happy, as in touch with their bodies, or as truly liberated as they thought they were or wished to be.

Yoga can be our space to make change and take the right action. It is a space where body acceptance can be realized, and it can also be a platform for amplifying marginalized voices. Practicing yoga strengthens our hearts so we can put in the real work of awakening. It is important to be able to accept that the people we love and respect, whose opinions we value, might not always agree with us. We are all, in some ways, exactly who we need as a hero in our lives.

INCLUSIVITY IN THE YOGA COMMUNITY

Conversations about inclusivity decide who gets to be well, elevated, and happy in society. People in positions of power ultimately determine who is deemed worthy of receiving care, rest, and support, who will literally have the space to breathe with ease. Yoga practice helps everyone access their whole selves. To truly make this practice inclusive, we have to be willing to have difficult conversations about privilege and its harmful effects.

Yoga asks each of us to step outside the boundaries of our comfort zone. This could be a form of tapas, or "moving into the fire." In a way, yoga is very confrontational. The practice asks us to face that with which we are unfamiliar or uncomfortable and ultimately come out the other side a little stronger for it. If we practice yoga regularly, many of us face this confrontation on a daily basis. Stepping out of your comfort zone is the only way to grow, both physically and emotionally. Yoga practice gives us the tools we need to step off the edge of familiarity and into more divergent points of view.

Ultimately, we must each ask ourselves how we can help create a space for everyone to safely explore the unfamiliar. From the language we use to the way we approach showing up in class, there are opportunities everywhere. The key is communication and moving out of a space of complacency into one of action. Small steps into the unknown are sometimes all it takes to inspire others to take that step out of their own comfort zone.

Yoga is a spiritual practice that represents the potential for equity and justice when people become their higher selves. Transformative justice can start on the yoga mat, but it will only be fully realized in its expression in the world. I have often been criticized for making yoga political, but it is impossible to be a yoga teacher and student today and not be socially engaged. The definition of yoga is evolving and expanding day by day. Being a yoga practitioner requires more from us than just doing our daily practice and forgetting about yoga for the rest of the day.

I want to take a moment to acknowledge the work of Wambui Njuguna-Räisänenin and Lashanna Small, who are at the leading edge of social justice work within the Ashtanga Yoga tradition. For those seeking to dive deeper into the intersection of yoga and social justice, I recommend looking into their work. Being a socially engaged yoga practitioner does not mean giving up on yoga or being angry and upset all the time. It means waking up in every moment of our lives. It means gaining new perspectives to enhance our practice and improve the emotional and spiritual well-being of the world in our own way.

Perhaps as more yoga studios engage in social justice and collective change, spiritual teachers and communities will find more ways to apply the insights from our various practices and teachings for the good of all. It should also be noted that different countries and cultures will have different expectations of and needs from a yoga space. The work of every yoga student begins with unlearning their old samskaras. Unlearning is a multipronged process of identifying the selective information and versions of history we have learned and making a conscious decision to question this education and seek out more knowledge. It isn't easy to rewire our brains to think differently about ourselves and our history, but it's a process we as yoga practitioners must begin.

Sitting with the uncomfortable, relearning what we think we know about our minds and our bodies—these are all elements of our yoga practice. Just as we practice holding ourselves accountable on the yoga mat, we can also practice holding ourselves accountable in our yoga communities. Progress often does not feel like progress. Working on the inner terrain of unlearning can feel murky and unsettling, but that does not mean it is not working. As always, we have to keep practicing.

Teaching yoga is many things that change depending on the requirements of the student that day and over time. It may simply be a few adjustments, help getting into an asana. It may be something more physically therapeutic. For new students, slowly learning the series, and for long-term students, deeper teachings of a spiritual nature and just occasionally a new asana. There is also the importance of the student's mental and emotional health to consider. As one gets to know a student better and discover their trials and tribulations, a teacher can adjust their style, information given, pranayama taught, spiritual teachings and other advice given.

—HAMISH HENDRY

4

Culture & Heritage

YOGA IS NOW more accessible than ever. No matter where you are starting your yoga journey—be it online or with a teacher—there is no reason for students or teachers to feel like they cannot find an authentic connection to the practice's roots.

Yoga is like a stream. The flow of the stream existed before the current era. As students and teachers, we step into the flow and interact with it. One day we will step out of the flow of yoga, but it will nevertheless keep flowing once we exit. Thinking of the history of yoga as a perpetually flowing stream is one way to understand what lineage represents. This requires us to have a multidimensional outlook, to look to the past and the future, and to be aware of where we are on the journey. Yoga lineage is not the type of lineage that involves genetics or bloodlines. The only qualification to enter a yoga lineage is to consciously and intentionally do the practice and integrate the lessons of yoga into your life.

Yoga is an intentional type of connection from teacher to student that can also be understood like the passing of a flame from one candle to another. The teacher is merely one whose spark of fire was ignited by someone else before. The teacher then lights the metaphorical candle of the student, who may one day pass the spark of ignition on to another. The flame keeps burning through each person who passes it on. When you devote yourself to yoga practice, you are not devoting yourself to your teacher but to the source from which the lineage originates.

While yoga is considered a devotional practice, we have to think about what we are actually devoting ourselves to. Ideally yoga promotes independence and self-responsibility. Unfortunately, sometimes devotion also runs the risk of promoting dependence and powerlessness. Devotion to yoga is about recognizing that the ideal of the practice is your highest self. When you encourage yourself to go deeper, understand more, and evolve, you are rising to the challenge of the practice. It may be helpful to reconceptualize lineage as a system that rejects control, authoritarianism, and suppression. Instead of yoga entrenching power hierarchies, we can think about how yoga uproots them. It frees the mind, which is a direct challenge to systemic oppression, while at the same time being a tradition steeped in history and culture. To complicate things further, the industrialization and capitalization of yoga skews the foundational bedrock of the practice as profit maximization can easily compromise its soul. And yet, yoga practice currently exists within the network of exchange that is our contemporary economy. Students pay for yoga classes, materials, and resources. Teachers are paid for their work and must sustain themselves. Producers of yoga products must be profitable in order to pay their labor force. The industry itself is unavoidable in our current socioeconomic structure. Industrialization, however, is something to watch in the burgeoning economy of yoga.

Mainstream yoga is a new trend in the West, spawning an endless sea of clothing lines and gimmicky classes with cute farm animals or beer to entice students to practice. The yoga practice of the West often brushes over the faith and history that is at work on the mat. It becomes the responsibility of every practitioner to learn more and create more space for other members of the yoga community. Of course, the responsibility falls to an even greater degree on all who would consider themselves yoga teachers and industry leaders in the yoga space.

Take a moment to reflect on your yoga practice. No matter where you are on your journey, you have put in a good amount of work to get here. The practice of yoga itself has come even further, surviving thousands of years in India through an unbroken succession of generations of yogis whose deeper intention to the spiritual path was unwavering. We share the path with the lineage of practitioners from centuries ago who have protected and preserved this practice so we may continue on its journey today. We each owe the ancient yogis an incalculable debt.

There is an invitation for every contemporary yoga student to be curious about the origin culture of yoga. Modern yogis can cultivate a sense of cultural appreciation for the practice through a respect for the cradle of yoga. To reclaim the wholeness of yoga, each student is charged with the task of respecting and honoring the origin culture of yoga. Students cannot rely on teachers to do it for them. That means yoga students can learn how to move away from cultural appropriation and embrace cultural appreciation. While there is no substitute for making the trip to India to study the practice as a way of honoring the roots of yoga, yoga students all over the world can learn to honor those roots without having to reinvent the spiritual path.

Once they have learned a bit about yoga's heritage, some students and teachers grow weary and hesitant, wishing to avoid cultural appropriation. That sense of caution may be a good thing if it challenges the assumptions of privilege. If you are a non-Indian yoga student, it is responsible to reflect on how your actions impact the ancient and established spiritual journey.

In yoga the idea of lineage is important, yet it is often misunderstood. Lineage is the ancestry of a tradition, the chain along which the teachings are passed from teacher to student. You might think of it as a line from teacher to student that transfers knowledge, but it's good to remember that it takes more than one point to make a line. A traditional metaphor for lineage is that it is like a tree branch. As you trace a branch back further and further, you discover new smaller branches shooting off the original— some straight, some angled to the side—but they all come together to form one branch that is part of one tree. In yoga when you can trace a similar pattern, it is a sign that the lineage is alive and healthy—you'll find the main branch of teachings with many teachers who each have their own interpretation and method for getting the basic ideas across— still connected to the branch but adding their own character.

—RICHARD FREEMAN and MARY TAYLOR

If you are a non-Indian yoga teacher, that reflection is not optional but mandatory. We must be encouraged to embark on true self-reflection and discover what it means to honor yoga's roots.

There is, in fact, a big difference between cultural *appropriation* and true cultural *appreciation*. Cultural appropriation occurs when a member of the dominant group of society uses aspects of a nondominant culture for personal gain. This often occurs at the expense of members of the non-dominant group. For example, non-Indian yoga teachers may appropriate Indian accents to appear more authentic, whereas Indian yoga teachers are often judged negatively for their accents in other situations.

The images presented in popular culture are often intimidating and fail to portray the story of yoga within India's historic past. There is a rich cultural heritage contained within the lineage that often gets edited out of popular how-to articles and quick guides to yoga. Deep, powerful teachings about subtle energy centers like the chakras or mudras get reduced to memes. Yoga is so much more than what we can find online. There is no substitute for finding a teacher whose life testifies to their commitment to yoga and studying with them in person over a long period of time.

While yoga practice relies on the dedication of teachers, it is important to remember that all teachers, even the great sages and rishis of times past, are fallible and imperfect, just like you and me. Learning needs a balance between a healthy notion of self-worth and humility. Finding this balance is a feat yoga students have to face more than once. Once we learn to recognize our teachers as ordinary human beings, a deeper level of learning can begin to take shape. Anyone placed on a pedestal of perfection will one day fall off and leave those who held them up as the standard disappointed. Worse than that, people who put others on high pedestals are more likely to hold themselves up to these same unattainable standards, which will only detract from spiritual growth. Through yoga practice, you are seeking a community with other human beings who are on this same path. When it comes to yoga teachers, they are simply farther along on this path.

Perhaps a good way of considering the authority of a yoga teacher is as one of deferential rather than absolute authority. If you consult Google Maps for directions, you trust the source for a period of time within reasonable standards. But if the map directs you to drive into the ocean, you will (hopefully) stop. Just because Google Maps knows the way, it doesn't mean the application is more intelligent or evolved than we are. Instead, the knowledge contained within the app is a tool for us to use on our journey. Much in the same way, we can think of teachers as holding a kind of spiritual map that can assist with our journey. We are going to get lost and stumble on this journey, and teachers are there to give us directions. They have the knowledge and forethought to lead us a little further, but they are not the absolute authorities over our practice. Every student's journey is fueled in some part by a teacher of some sort, even if the relationship is virtual or remote. The authority of the yoga teacher is rooted in the community and the sacred relationship between the teacher and student.

Every yoga student needs a teacher. Even if someone thinks they are self-taught, no one ever really ventures into the spiritual journey totally alone. Not everyone can travel to India in search of a yoga guru. In Sanskrit, the teacher-student relationship is called the *guru-shishya* relationship, and it is a key aspect of the yoga journey. Finding a teacher who supports your vulnerability and your agency can be challenging, but we all must strive to find someone who works best to support our practice.

Questioning or perhaps reenvisioning the guru-shishya model with the intersection of yoga and social justice in mind is where many members of yoga community find themselves today. Many Ashtanga Yoga students and teachers were forced into a period of reflection in the aftermath of the revelations of the sexual assaults committed by K. Pattabhi Jois. Rather than wait for the perfect solution, teachers and students showed up to guide each other side by side. In many ways the Ashtanga community is still processing the evolution of the lineage. Where it all lands will perhaps only be seen clearly in retrospect. Meanwhile, there is no need to wait for the perfect leaders to show up or to judge those who are in place. We can lift up those who are leading in an inspiring way for us. Ashtanga Yoga is a paradox right now. In some sense there is no central governing body to provide checks and balances. However, Ashtanga Yoga has a clear lineage holder and a system of authority centralized around the Ashtanga Institutes in Mysore, India. Perhaps for now, we can operate both inside and outside the system. Maybe it is possible to feel grace while sitting at the guru's feet and simultaneously question the guru model.

DECOLONIZING THE LINEAGE

The lineage of yoga is a sacred key to our practice. Unfortunately, the way yoga is packaged up and delivered today—especially in the West—can have an impact on our personal and individual connections to the practice. Some would think that the lineage is just postural by looking at contemporary yoga literature, but asanas alone are not the essence of lineage or the essence of yoga practice.

While asana is a part of yoga practice, it is just one element of the faith and the lineage that many people of South Asian descent know as their culture and heritage. The history of modern postural yoga has been much debated, and there are certainly historical inaccuracies that we cannot deny. Nevertheless, there is ample evidence that points toward a verification of yoga's ancient past. The impact that British occupation had on the spiritual community of yoga within India must also be included in any discussion of yoga history. Up until the British colonization, there was a new yoga treatise published about every one hundred years or so by an

Yoga has never been just one thing; it is alive and changing all the time. Yoga, like many indigenous practices, has now become globalized and commercialized. Many of the spiritual practitioners who promulgate various teachings that originate from Black and brown communities lack the immersive depth in the culture of origin to truly teach with nuance and subtlety. Instead, under the banner of Westernized principles, the barriers to entry into the sacred domain of spiritual practice are removed, and practices that were once reserved for the most respected and experienced members of a community to teach are now available for all in the form of a two-hundred–hour Yoga Teacher Training. In one sense, this is a kind of liberation (clearly sharing knowledge and opportunity with everyone is a good thing for a spiritual practice). In another sense, this is a kind of disregard for the seriousness and gravity that entry into spiritual societies once required. Westerners keep adapting yoga however they like and teaching it without an understanding of why these very precious spiritual practices were never meant to be taught by just anyone. What all students and teachers of yoga need to remember is that this is the cultural history and legacy of a people who have suffered at the hands of white colonial ancestors.

—JOSEPH ARMSTRONG and
EDGAR NAVARRO ARCHILA

When we walk into a yoga room anyplace in the world and we meet the person leading the class, remember that it would be a miracle if the person in front of you is an enlightened being, a Sat Guru. Most likely you can optimistically expect a human being much like yourself, who hopefully has enough experience and knowledge about the yoga methods and tradition to guide you a bit further along the path than where you are already. Yet as yoga has hit mainstream and pursuing this ancient discipline simply as a professional vocation is now common, even that is not a given. In a best-case scenario, this can lead the yoga student down a path of true seeking and constructive discernment, while a traumatic experience of personal boundaries shattered is also within possibilities. Surrender is considered the optimal state for true yogic learning, yet encountering a true guru who can embody such superhuman responsibility is considered more than rare. If we choose to surrender ourselves in some fashion to a yoga teacher, master, or guru, whether in the hope of a new asana, a more joyful mind, enlightenment, or an itty bit of happiness, we can do ourselves a big favor by recognizing that 99 percent of the time we are simply standing in front of another human being, flawed and amazing, just like ourselves. If we can allow ourselves to see the apparent hero yoga authority simply as a human being whose knowledge of the subject exceeds our own, then perhaps we can find

▶

accomplished yogi. But during the time of the British Raj, yoga was suppressed as an antiestablishment practice of rebellion (which it is!). As such, yogis and gurus went into hiding, and very few new treatises on the practice were published until India's independence. It has even been argued that Patanjali's Yoga Sutras were crafted by the British to be the canonical text of yoga because of their emphasis on nonviolence as the foundations of yoga. There is much to say about the history of British rule in India that exceeds the scope of this book, and I encourage interested students to continue their studies with the many resources available today. We can spark the seed of inquiry that may help decolonize our view of yoga and perhaps more as well.

Decolonizing is not just a trendy buzzword. Instead, it is crucial to reflect on and unpack the historical implications of colonization and how it manifests now in history, media, and the wellness community. Colonization is a kind of whitewashing of culture that removes aspects of the origin culture that the colonizers deem unpalatable. Colonization and cultural appropriation go hand in hand. Look for both to be present when Sanskrit words are removed from yoga class and replaced by English terms that have no reference to the original Sanskrit. Or when Sanskrit mantras and invocations are erased and loud pop music takes their place. Students miss out on the true essence of what the yoga scriptures teach us, and those students who follow us will continue to be limited by this narrowed perspective. We can use our yoga practice as a tool to dismantle the structure of colonization in our minds. We can listen to traditional teachers of Indian origin, give minority voices a platform, and step out of the echo chamber of the colonized mindset.

Each of us, as yoga students, has the responsibility to honor the lineage of yoga and maintain our agency as yogis. By educating ourselves and seeking out diverse voices and perspectives, we can move away from the colonized perspective and break down any of the unconscious barriers in our own minds that could be translating into our practice. We can appreciate and engage with these tools of spiritual devotion and realization without harming the culture of origin. Truly inspired students can learn how to immerse themselves within the origin culture of India.

Yoga is an ancient practice passed on from teacher to student over millennia, and the tradition of yoga is kept alive by the students—people like you and me—taking time to get on the mat and practice every day. The culture of yoga is essential to the student's journey, and everyone who practices yoga is in a sort of debt to the practice itself. We owe it to ourselves and the future generation of yogis to protect and honor the culture and teachings.

What about Namaste?

Almost every yoga class begins or ends with *Namaste*. While it is at home within a yoga class, this word has been appropriated across the West on T-shirts and wine glasses, used as a catcall and to sell mimosas at brunch.

While people may say this is all done in jest and is harmless, it's more than that. Hearing or reading "Namaslay" or "Nama-stay-in-bed" or other such wordplay is, at best, based in ignorance. Using namaste outside of its true meaning may create confusion for the incoming generation of yoga practitioners who may not know any better.

Namaste, sometimes seen as *Namaskar* and *Namaskaram*, is a customary, noncontact form of respectfully greeting and honoring another person or group at any time of the day or night. Used throughout India and many parts of Asia, most Western yoga students first hear this word at the beginning and end of many yoga classes. The gesture associated with the word is called Anjali Mudra (Salutation Seal), which refers to the divine offering held in the cavity formed between the hands and given as a form of worship.

Namaste usually includes a type of *pranam*, or slight bow, and in India there are many types of pranams or prostrations, of which this is merely one.

Namaste combines the word *namas*, which means "bow," "reverential salutation," or "obeisance," and the second-person pronoun *te*, which means "to you." Some common translations include "I bow to the Divine in you," and "The Divine in me recognizes the Divine in you." The word can be found in Vedic literature, including the *Rig Veda* and *Atharva Veda Samhita*; in post-Vedic texts such as Mahabharata, and in ancient Indus Valley civilization artwork and Hindu temples. Namaste can be used as a respectful greeting and to express gratitude toward another person. Toward a deity, it can express deeper spiritual devotion.

Bear in mind that this chapter does not seek to define the places where the usage of Namaste is acceptable but is instead meant to educate regarding the word's origins and traditional usage. The last thing I would want to do is create a Namaste police force charged with cancelling yoga teachers who fail to comply with a set of diction and syntax rules. Remember that cultural appropriation happens when the dominant group of society takes pieces from nondominant cultures for its own use and profits from them in a way that is inaccessible to the nondominant culture. With this in mind, we as students of yoga would do well to study the true meaning of Namaste, its etymology and pronunciation, and how appropriation can dilute its impact on our yoga journey.

As students of yoga, we strive to find a balance and educate ourselves and those around us to respect yoga culture without appropriating it. We are encouraged to move into a space of knowledge and not just practice. Yoga gives us the spiritual tools to move away from ignorance and into the truth, and it is through our practice that we can not only educate ourselves but also teach others the true roots of the culture and the practice.

Hinduphobia

There is a reason that Western culture appropriates a word like *Namaste* without fully understanding its meaning. Many of us, myself included,

the appropriate degree of surrender and open ourselves up to the right level of learning in a healthy manner. When we learn from yoga teachers and masters, it is advisable to gradually build mutual trust, trusting our own gut feeling of healthy physical, emotional, and spiritual boundaries. The concept of complete surrender is meant only for the Sat Guru, and they are more than rare to come by. Just as we would not give our friendship easily to any random person, perhaps we can be discriminating in our choice of teacher, guide, and guru as well.

—TIM FELDMANN

We can absolutely challenge Western notions of how we should practice, what the space should feel like, what parampara ("the lineage passed from teacher to student") is and can BE. We can also honor yoga's Eastern origins, while calling into accountability some of its nuances that might not be so innocuous. The idea of a decolonized yoga space is simply a place where we can acknowledge the various identity politics and privilege dynamics that exist in the world and still seek to combat them, not by pretending that they don't exist, but by confronting them with accountability and action, valuing true and impactful inclusion of marginalized communities, extending ourselves and each other grace when we falter (because it is inevitable that we will), and moving forward as a community, a *real* "sangha" stronger BECAUSE of the ways in which we vary, not in spite of it.

—KIRA WILLIAMS BOUWER

often first engage with yoga through a colonized lens. We sign up for a class at our gym or watch a video about yoga and never realize the spiritual experience or rich cultural history that is intricately woven into the practice. What has been marketed in the West as a fitness package is so much more than physical exercise. Yoga is a philosophy of life, and yoga philosophy is one of the major components of the Hindu faith. We cannot remove the truth about yoga's connection to the Hindu dharma. It should also be noted that the word *Hindu* itself might be seen as a colonized word. Some South Indian scholars have argued that the culture of India's past is actually better defined as the followers of the Sanatana dharma. Most people in the West, who lack the subtle references to India's spiritual legacy, merely understand Indian spiritual teaching as Hindu and sometimes perpetuate fear and anxiety around a foreign culture.

Fear around the Hindu faith can result in Hinduphobia and the erasure of the Hindu culture, both of which have appeared in the yoga community. There is tremendous trepidation in some faith-based communities in the West around Hindu culture. Despite that fear, yoga's popularity has created a schism in some places where many people like the asanas but remain hesitant about embracing Hindu culture. While it may seem incredible, there are certain faith leaders who proclaim that backbending, yogic breathing techniques, and other parts of yoga practice open students to demonic possession. These faith leaders forbid members of their communities from attending yoga classes. For people living in communities where fear-based paradigms dominate, it may be tempting to simply remove all elements of India from yoga and just keep the poses. This, however, would be a disservice to truthfulness and a heinous act of cultural appropriation. Hindu erasure is manifest in language barriers and accessibility. When yoga teachers remove or consciously refrain from including Indian references, Sanskrit words, and other key identifiers of Hindu dharma in their classes, they devalue the origin culture of yoga. Of course, we are all on a journey as teachers and students, and we may have every intention of learning the Sanskrit names of the poses but simply haven't done it yet. This does not mean that yoga is not for non-Indian students or teachers. The practice deserves students and teachers who are respectful of its history and are willing to step out of their comfort zone to practice in a way that is culturally aware. Yoga practitioners who want to do the right thing and practice yoga respectfully need to move forward working with their own biases, subconscious or otherwise. If you become a yoga teacher, then you are responsible for learning the roots of your practice. You deserve the experience of cultural immersion, and a trip to India to study the beginnings of the spiritual path will only help you gain a new perspective of this ancient practice. "Exotifying" and fetishizing a foreign culture without truly understanding its history and context engenders harm. To make the effort to learn is a sign of respect. You have the power to drive the narrative, and if you are erasing Sanskrit from your practice, it has an impact far beyond the confines of your mat.

The Spiritual Responsibility of the Yoga Student

All the sacred teachings from the spiritual tradition of India have been passed on with great responsibility from one generation to the next. To step into the lineage, all that is required is to practice yoga as a spiritual path in every moment of your life, to the best of your ability.

The spiritual readiness of the student is very important when it comes to taking the first step on this journey. Not everyone is willing to commit themselves to the practice even if they feel a pull toward it. Every student needs to evaluate whether yoga practice is really the right path for them. To commit to the practice is to commit to yoga as a spiritual path for one's entire life.

This is not a workout routine, although it can help you lose weight and improve your health. It also is not a trend that you can drop once it is no longer trendy. Yoga is a spiritual tradition that has been practiced for many centuries and passed on from generation to generation. Practicing yoga means joining the chain of thousands of practitioners who came before you. To step onto this path is not to step lightly or inconsequentially. Physical adaptations can be made for the asanas, but the spiritual and mental adjustments that need to be made for your spiritual growth must come from within.

Yoga is for the student who is willing to show up regularly and put in the work. You are the only one who can bring yourself to the mat every day, and you are also the only one who can carry the practice with you in your daily life.

Patanjali's teachings say that we must practice yoga without a break, but that doesn't necessarily mean being on the mat every hour of every day. Instead, we live the teachings of yoga when we let the moral and ethical precepts of the practice infuse every part of our lives, from our speech to our actions to how we participate in society. Reflecting on our own identity within the context of yoga helps us situate ourselves within the larger context of yoga, colonization, and history. I am a white-passing, multiethnic person, and my ancestry has been a source of personal contemplation and discovery. The colonial imprint plays a big role in our construction of the world and is the foundational paradigm of our worldview. There are so many presuppositions about who has access to power, privilege, and opportunities. There is a strong intersection between wealth and skin color. The existing power hierarchies have impacted yoga's global reach. To a large degree, yoga has been promulgated in spaces of privilege throughout the global wellness culture outside India.

Sometimes it may seem like there is a lack of connection between getting on the mat in the service of liberation and the work of liberating every

In a sense, many Ashtangis are well educated in a liberal and individualistic reading of the yoga philosophy. "We are all one" can be accommodated like this: "We live in a racist country. I am sorry for that. I do my practice and hope it will stop someday." A spiritual path is not a matter of an individual being enlightened. It is not the victory of an individual soul. It is not a matter of an individual getting better and better and performing, mastering more and more. Controlling, controlling. After all, the winner takes all. A spiritual path outside this individualistic view is to realize deeply that there is no separation and that our work should also be collective and social. No action is an action as well, Krishna teaches Arjuna. Yoga, like everything, is political. It is a living tradition, something we construct anew all the time. And a living tradition may change too.

—MARCOS SILVA

human being. There is no way we can say that we truly want all beings to be happy unless we are at least willing to make it accessible for every being to be able to get on a mat and actually do the practice. If the image of yoga globally becomes edified in institutions that idolize Eurocentric ideologies, we will perpetuate the harm of colonization. If we can connect the work we do on the mat with unpacking the stuff within ourselves, then liberation can truly be for all.

There is a discrepancy between the origin culture of yoga and the dominant culture of Western wellness spaces. We must approach the practice of yoga in solidarity with the most oppressed communities of the world. It can feel daunting to think about where we go from here and envision what the new dream of a loving world looks like.

Perhaps it is about getting practical about ethics, changing what gets taught in yoga classes, and examining the way in which power and privilege enslave us. Dismantling systems of oppression is not something that is done for someone else, but it is done because our own liberation depends on it. Maybe we will find a way toward an actively engaged front and center where justice and truth exist in a way that is kind, nourishing, and fun.

Seeing more diversity within the student body, teachers, and people in positions of power feels like a step in the right direction. Perhaps there is a way we can learn to confront things without confronting each other. Maybe that will come when we are able to accept all the parts of ourselves that do not fit the mold of the dominant narrative. Imagine if we could let yoga be a space where no one needs to attenuate who they are to fit in the room. Every body—big, small, old, young, Black, brown, disabled, queer—is truly welcome. All anyone needs to do is practice. The *Hatha Yoga Pradipika* says that yoga cannot be attained by intellectual study, adopting certain behaviors or modes of dress, or talking about the practice. Instead, it says, "Constant practice alone is the secret of success" (1:66). This book is about giving every inspired student the tools they need to continue their practice.

Complex asanas can be fun, but they cannot take us away from the work of excavating deeper layers of ourselves. As we reposition ourselves away from what a homogenous view of a yoga room looks like and realign toward a heterogenous and inclusive space, yoga becomes truly more accessible.

The new yoga room is not about prioritizing and valuing advanced asanas where the teacher always knows what is right. A truly inclusive space is integrated across many intersections. Maybe the yoga center doesn't have to be yoga-only. Yoga centers can turn into community centers that hold space for difficult conversations, philosophical study, and more. Maybe there is a rhizomatic yoga community that will emerge and flourish and redefine all the norms.

Yoga has saved the lives of so many people. People who spend ten or twenty years—or a whole lifetime—practicing rely on their practice to ground their lives. Living a healthier life is multilayered. Self-care and self-healing go hand in hand with collective care and collective healing. Justice, like trauma, lives in the body. Understanding how justice lives in the somatic experience of the cells is the basis of liberation in yoga.

PRESERVING WHAT IS SACRED ABOUT YOGA

You are attracted to the goodness in yoga by the goodness that is within yourself. Everything you have achieved and accomplished so far is a result of all your efforts and dedication to the practice. Give yourself the validation you deserve for coming to the mat every day. It is your effort that keeps you moving on this path, and it is this same effort that preserves the tradition of the practice.

You choose yoga (and yourself) every time you commit to your practice. Every time you sit on the mat, it's a choice you consciously make to continue this journey and live your own yoga. Like all living things, yoga practice must be nurtured. Our journey on this path is a lesson in kindling and rekindling the fire that inspired us to take up yoga in the first place.

Every student that comes onto the path of yoga has the opportunity to experience real peace and real happiness, and I hope I inspire you as much as you inspire me. It can be hard to make this commitment, but I know we all love yoga enough to keep trying and keep practicing. The tradition of yoga is in our hands as students. Thousands of generations of yogis have come before us, setting the groundwork and giving us a path to start on. Now it is our turn to set the foundation for the next generation of yogis. Let us be good ancestors in the lineage of yoga.

Irrespective of place of birth, either East or West, the inclination for healthy and peaceful life or spirituality is there in all yoga aspirants. So once they start practicing, it further improves the sattva guna like Sage Patanjali describes as "sattva shuddhi" (2.41). So equal-minded people can come together, making a platform to know, share, practice, and grow. Like there is an association for business or medicine, associations in the yoga field can help the seekers, practitioners, and teachers. Yoga brings transformation to bring about a unity through equality.

—DR. PAVITHRA KUMAR

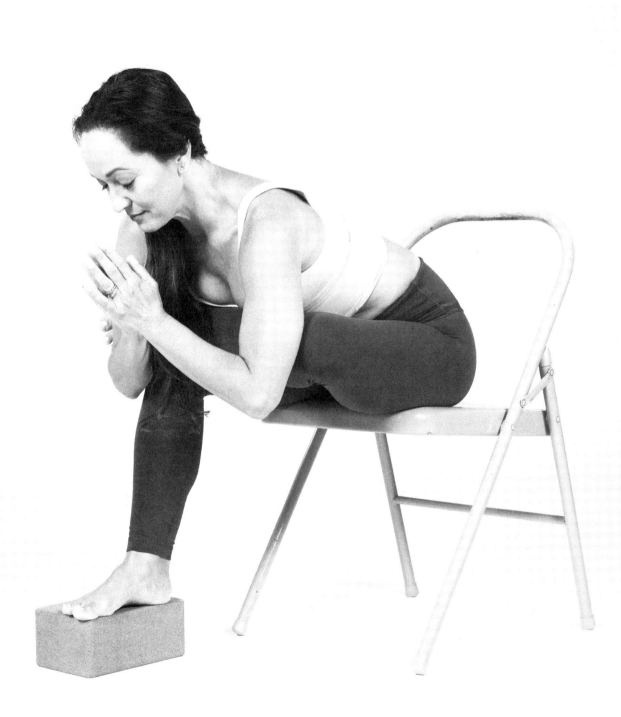

PART TWO

Accessible Practice

WHILE THIS BOOK is no substitute for working directly with a qualified teacher, my hope is that the variations and adaptations will lead the way for students and teachers alike in their journey toward accessibility. Ashtanga Yoga is truly for everyone, or at least it can be, if we put in the effort to renovate the mechanics of the practice. These variations of the asanas are for you at different stages of your life and for your students and friends as they work on the foundations of the asanas. Some asanas will be appropriate as alternatives to practice during pregnancy and postpartum. Others will open a door to intimidating asanas for students who want to explore new avenues of the practice. But, more than anything, these variations of the asanas are meant to shed light on the path of practice, to help redefine what asana practice is and what it can be. Instead of the body of students changing to meet one standard, it is the asana that changes to meet the diversity of students. Not everyone needs to practice yoga, but yoga needs to be adapted to every student who truly wants to practice.

A student with a neurodegenerative disease recently joined a class of mine. It was inspiring to see how much she benefited from the practice and how necessary it was to adapt the practice to better suit her needs. The practice of yoga is a relationship between teacher and student; between mind and body; and between past, present, and future. Just as any relationship evolves over time, so too must the practice if it is to thrive and remain useful for all who seek its benefits.

Compassion and empathy spring from true understanding of the needs and feelings of others. Without accessible variations of all the asanas, the benefits of this practice may remain relegated to an elite few with a certain set of physical characteristics. That was never the intention of yoga. As you explore adaptations for the asanas in the Second Series, be careful not to think of these as "easy." Instead, respect the integrity of the practice and use these variations to support the inner work. Respecting the students who show up is the core of teaching, and the asanas are tools to facilitate each student's journey. If the focus shifts to respecting the asana above the student, then we have veered off the path of compassion and awakening. Each student is on their own unique path, and the asanas are adapted to the needs of each student, but the adaptations do not dilute the impact of the asanas themselves. Yoga is hard work, and that remains true whether the practice is supported by a chair, a block, a yoga mat, a teacher's assist, or any other means.

The instructions for the variations of the asana previously covered in *Power of Ashtanga Yoga I* and *II* will not be repeated. Instead, emphasis will be placed on instructions for the adaptive versions of the asanas.

5

Sun Salutations

THE SPARK OF THE DIVINE, represented as the sun, is contained within every particle of energy in the universe, including you and me. When we practice Surya Namaskars (Sun Salutations), we are acknowledging not only the power of the sun in a physical sense within our solar system but the spark of the Divine within ourselves and all beings. The Sun Salutations ignite a kind of alchemical metamorphosis of the body and mind during the flow of the practice. The light of God illuminates the yoga practitioner with an inner glow, and it begins with the Sun Salutations. It is not only a physical warm-up but also a time to concentrate the mind and focus the spirit.

Surya Namaskar A (Sun Salutation A)

The first Sun Salutation sequence begins and ends in Samasthitih (Equal Standing) and marks the beginning of the practice. The internal solar fire is cultivated along with a recognition of the external light that the sun provides to start each day. Each of the movements outlined here is held for one breath except the last Adho Mukha Svanasana (Downward-Facing Dog Pose), which is held for five breaths. While each pose is usually coordinated with either an inhalation or an exhalation, it may be necessary or advisable to add an extra breath where necessary to more safely enter and exit a pose. Always coordinate breath with movement. Repeat this sequence three to seven times or until the body is sufficiently warmed up.

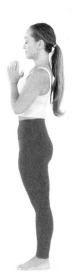

Figure 5.1

Samasthitih (Equal Standing)

Samasthitih is the alpha and the omega, the beginning and the end, the balanced stillness that harkens back to the mythical origins of yoga. When Sanskrit numbers are counted in a traditional Ashtanga Yoga practice, the count derives from starting and ending every single pose in Samasthitih. Associated more with the space between breaths than either inhalation or exhalation, there is no traditional or specific breathing pattern associated with the pose. Yet, there is both mystery and intelligence contained in this asana. Sometimes called the blueprint for every other pose, Samasthitih is said to represent the Divine emptiness from which all things spring forth and the cosmic abyss into which all things dissolve. A qualified and experienced teacher can make an accurate assessment of physical ailments, postural misalignments, and other issues that may present during yoga practice simply by astutely observing a student in Samasthitih. Sometimes confused with Tadasana (Mountain Pose), which is an asana in the Fourth Series/Advanced B Section of Ashtanga Yoga, Samasthitih is more like a standing meditation than other yoga poses. Representative of the state of active nondoing, it is also a call to the present moment and a command to begin the practice of yoga. Hidden within the call to presence are references to the Sanskrit word *atha* ("now") that marks the beginning of Patanjali's Yoga Sutras and indicates the spiritual readiness of the yoga practitioner. Every dedicated Ashtanga Yoga student feels the clarion call to step onto their mats and start the journey when they hear their teacher call out "Samasthitih." This pose is also the traditional place where the Opening and Closing Prayers are done (see "Appendix: Invocations" on page 222). The main image in this section shows the hands together, eyes closed, and the head slightly turned down to indicate the posture appropriate for prayer, while the photos that follow show the posture appropriate to commence practice. Now, let us begin.

CHAIR VARIATION

Start off seated on a chair. Shift the hips slightly forward to pivot into the fronts of the hip joints. Align the feet hip-width apart and plant the feet firmly on the ground. Lift the center of the chest, draw the muscles of the lower abdomen in toward the spine, and gently place the hands on the thighs. Gaze forward or toward the nose.

If the chair is used as a support, then start from standing instead. Place the chair in front of the body so that the seat of the chair is about an arm's length away. Align the feet hip-width apart, firmly plant the soles of the feet on the ground, and lift up from the arches. Engage the inner edges of the quadriceps and connect the legs into the pelvic floor. Draw the muscles of the pelvic floor upward and the muscles of the lower abdomen in toward the spine, allow the ribs to gently move upward to create space between the ribs and the hips, root the tips of the shoulder blades down the back, and let the arms hang by the sides of the torso. Extend upward through the crown of the head and gaze forward or toward the nose.

Figure 5.2

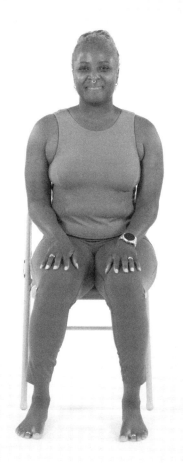

Figure 5.3

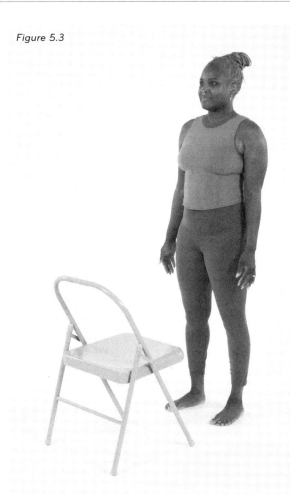

STANDING VARIATION

Align the bases of the big toes toward each other and align the feet accordingly. Sometimes it can be helpful to leave a little space between the heels. Place two blocks slightly ahead of the feet, shoulder-width apart. Plant the soles of the feet on the ground and lift up from the arches. Engage the inner edges of the quadriceps and connect the legs into the pelvic floor. Avoid squeezing the inner thighs or tightening anywhere in the body too much. Draw the muscles of the pelvic floor upward and the muscles of the lower abdomen in toward the spine, allow the ribs to gently move upward to create space between the ribs and the hips, root the tips of the shoulder blades down the back, and let the arms hang by the sides of the torso. Extend upward through the crown of the head and gaze forward or toward the nose.

Figure 5.4

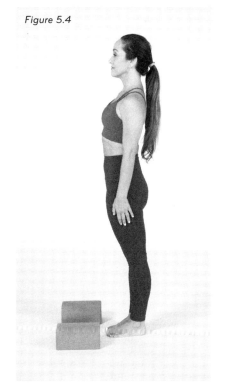

Figure 5.5

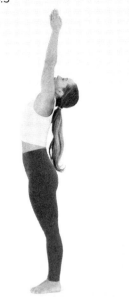

Ekam (One) and Nava (Nine)

CHAIR VARIATION

There are two ways to use the chair to support the practice of Sun Saluta-tions. Using the chair as a support instead of reaching all the way down to the floor in standing is a good adaptation for students who can bear some weight on their arms but have a hard time getting up from and down to the floor. Practicing the entire Sun Salutation sequence from the chair is better for students who have a hard time getting up and down from a seated position. Either way, find what works best to support your practice and continue to explore different variations.

Start off standing facing the seat of the chair to use the chair as a replace-ment for the floor. Separate the feet hip-width apart or place the feet together, whatever feels better for balance. Engage the muscles of the pelvic floor, draw the muscles of the lower abdomen in toward the spine, and lift the ribs away from the hips. Inhale and externally rotate the shoulders to lift the arms. Draw the elbows in toward the center line of the body and gently gaze upward (see fig. 5.6). If there is any strain in the neck, gaze forward.

Figure 5.6

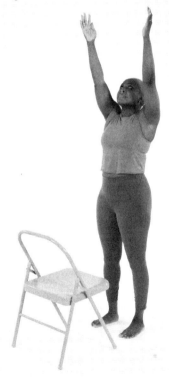

Start off seated in the chair to practice the entire sequence from this situation. Pivot slightly forward so the weight rests in the center of the seat of the chair. Align the feet hip-width apart and root down into the legs to ground the body. Engage the muscles of the pelvic floor, draw the muscles of the lower abdomen in toward the spine, and lift the ribs away from the hips. Inhale, externally rotate the shoulders to lift the arms, and lean for-ward into the hip creases. Draw the elbows in toward the center line of the body and gently gaze upward (see fig. 5.7). If there is any strain in the neck, gaze forward.

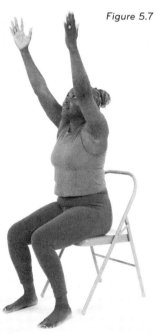

Figure 5.7

OTHER OPTIONS

Explore whether placing both the hands and the feet together is appropriate for the body. If not, try the same alignment outlined in the first Chair Variation.

Dwe (Two) and Astau (Eight) Uttanasana (Standing Forward Fold)

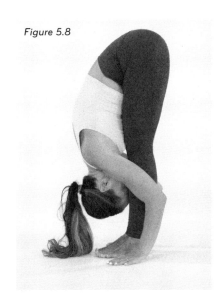

Figure 5.8

CHAIR VARIATION

Exhale and fold forward. Pivot at the hip joints, maintaining the muscular activation of the pelvic floor and lower abdomen. Firm the quadriceps to support the legs. Reach the hands down toward the seat of the chair and relax the neck (see fig. 5.9). Gaze either down or toward the nose.

Continuing from the seated position, exhale and pivot forward. Shift the body weight even more forward on the seat of the chair, and flex the hips to fold the torso as close to the thighs as possible. Engage the quadriceps to support the legs and ground the body. Place the hands on the knees and relax the head (see fig. 5.10). Gaze either down or toward the nose.

OTHER OPTIONS

Try bending the knees to fold forward or placing the hands on blocks on each side of the feet instead of the chair (see fig. 5.11).

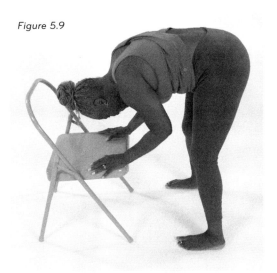

Figure 5.9

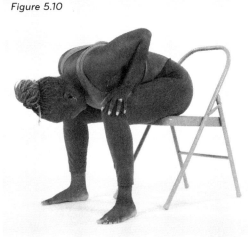

Figure 5.10

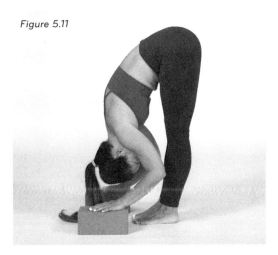

Figure 5.11

Figure 5.12

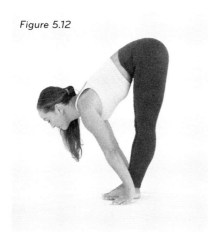

Trini (Three) and Sapta (Seven)

CHAIR VARIATION

Inhale and shift a little weight forward onto the hands. Lengthen the spine and send the center of the sternum up and forward. Draw the shoulder blades down the back, and gently activate the back muscles (see fig. 5.13). Remain vigilant about keeping the muscles of the pelvic floor and lower abdomen drawn in to support the spine in this slight spinal extension. Gaze forward or toward the nose.

Inhale and lengthen the spine. Send the center of the sternum up and forward. Draw the shoulder blades down the back, and gently activate the back muscles (see fig. 5.14). Remain vigilant about keeping the muscles of the pelvic floor and lower abdomen drawn in to support the spine in this slight spinal extension. Gaze forward or toward the nose.

Figure 5.13

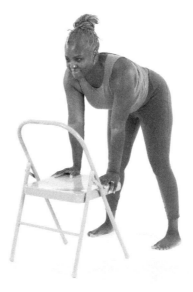

Figure 5.14

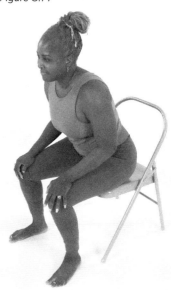

Figure 5.15

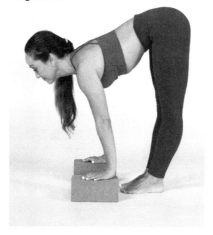

OTHER OPTIONS

Inhale and slide the hands up along the shinbones to create space. Or try keeping the hands on the blocks as the spine lifts away from the thighs (see fig. 5.15).

Chatuari (Four)
The Chaturanga Dandasana
(Four-Limbed Staff Pose)

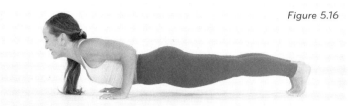

Figure 5.16

CHAIR VARIATION

Exhale and step the legs back to Kumbhakasana (Plank Pose) with the hands resting on the seat of the chair. This is deceptively hard, so walk back slowly (see fig. 5.17). Be sure the chair is set securely on the floor. Try placing the chair against a wall or on top of a sticky mat if it slides. Continue the exhalation, and bend the elbows when the shoulders and core feel strong enough to bear the weight of the body (see fig. 5.18)

Exhale and lift the arms off the thighs and push out into the air. Firm the muscles of the abdomen and engage the muscles of the shoulder girdle. Strengthen the quadriceps and connect into the feeling of strength throughout the whole body (see fig. 5.19). Explore bending the elbows to mimic the action of a push-up for an extra dose of strength (see fig. 5.20). Gaze forward or toward the nose.

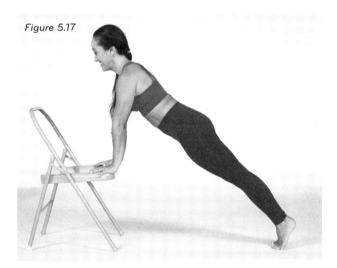

Figure 5.17

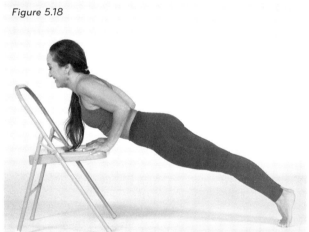

Figure 5.18

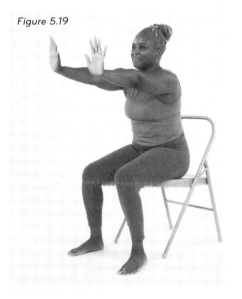

Figure 5.19

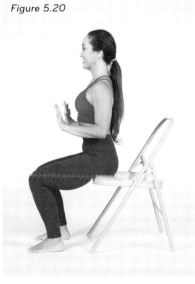

Figure 5.20

OTHER OPTIONS

Explore variations of Kumbhakasana as an alternative to Chaturanga Dandasana. Marjaryasana (Cat Pose) is also a good substitute and can be added to the sequence so that Bitilasana (Cow Pose) follows. Exhale and step back onto the hands and knees. Align the knees hip-width apart and the hands shoulder-width apart. Rotate the tailbone under and curl the spine into flexion. Stack the shoulders as much in line with the wrists and hands as possible. Tuck the head under and gaze toward the nose or the navel (see fig. 5.21).

Try placing a bolster under the body for support when lowering down from Kumbhakasana to Chaturanga Dandasana (see fig. 5.22). This allows the body to hold the pose without stressing the joints. If this feels comfortable, try lowering all the way down to the ground without the bolster and allowing the floor to support the body in the pose. If the wrists are sore, try Makara Adho Mukha Svanasana (Dolphin Plank Pose) as an alternative. Place the hands on two blocks aligned shoulder-width apart in Kumbhakasana. Firm the muscles of the pelvic floor and abdomen, bend the knees, and stabilize the shoulder girdle and upper back. Exhale and slowly lower to push-up position (see fig. 5.23). If this feels good, try keeping the knees off the ground when lowering from Kumbhakasana (see fig. 5.24). Eventually consider removing the blocks as strength builds throughout the body.

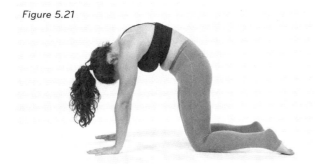

Figure 5.21

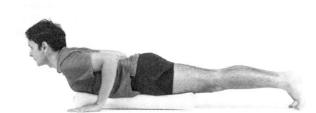

Figure 5.22

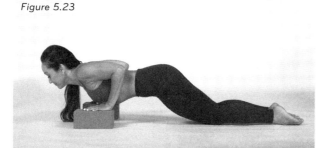

Figure 5.23

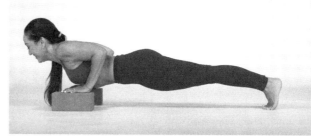

Figure 5.24

Panca (Five) Urdhva Mukha Svanasana (Upward-Facing Dog Pose)

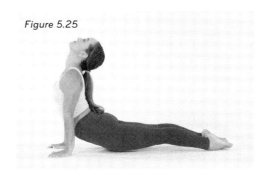

Figure 5.25

CHAIR VARIATION

Inhale and gently draw the chest up and forward, keeping the arms resting on the seat of the chair. Straighten the arms if they are bent. Gently arch the spine and activate the legs. Maintain the same foot position as in Kumbhakasana, or roll the toes over and point the feet (be sure the chair is well placed and will not slide for this option). Lift each vertebra away from the next to create space along the spinal axis. Engage the back muscles and pelvic floor. Draw the muscles of the lower abdomen in toward the spine. Expand the rib cage, and draw the shoulder blades down the spine. Gently reach the sternum and neck up and forward. Align the shoulders either on top of or just behind the wrists, and root down into the hands (see fig. 5.26). Gaze up or toward the nose.

Inhale and place the hands facing down on the thighs toward the knees. Gently arch the spine, lift the sternum up and forward, and turn the face about forty-five degrees up. Allow the elbows to bend slightly, and draw the shoulder blades down the back (see fig. 5.27). Maintain activation of the pelvic floor. Gaze up or toward the nose.

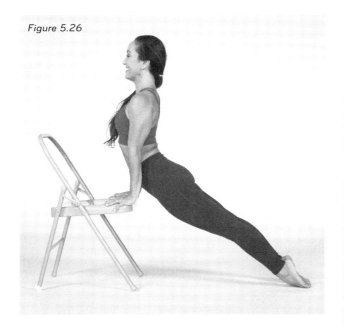

Figure 5.26

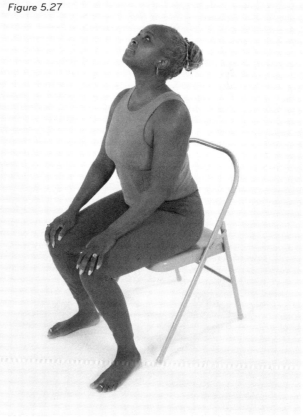

Figure 5.27

OTHER OPTIONS

Continuing from the hands-and-knees variation of Kumbhakasana, follow the breath to move from Marjaryasana to Bitilasana. Inhale and gently arch the spine. Lift each vertebra away from the next to create space along the spinal axis. Engage the back muscles and pelvic floor. Draw the muscles of the lower abdomen in toward the spine. Expand the rib cage, and draw the shoulder blades down the spine. Gently reach the sternum and neck up and forward. Align the shoulders either on top of or just behind the wrists, and root down into the hands (see fig. 5.28). Gaze up or toward the nose.

Bhujangasana (Cobra Pose) is a great alternative to Urdhva Mukha Svanasana. Allow the thighs to rest comfortably on the floor. Place the elbows forward of the shoulders, and draw the shoulder blades down the back. Inhale while lifting the ribs away from the hips, engaging the back muscles, and lifting along the center line of the body from the base of the spine up and out through the top of the head. Avoid craning the neck back. Soften the glutes but keep the thighs firm. Gaze toward the nose.

If the neck is sore, try gazing forward in Urdhva Mukha Svanasana (see fig. 5.29). If the back needs more space, try placing a block under each hand to give the lower back and legs more space (see fig. 5.30). If the body needs more support but is ready to move on from Bhujangasana, try keeping the bolster under the thighs for Urdhva Mukha Svanasana (see fig. 5.31).

Figure 5.28

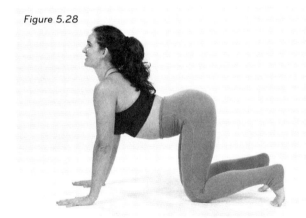

Figure 5.29

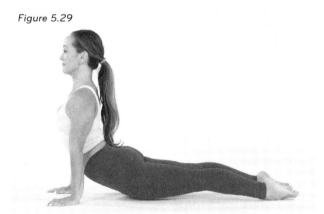

Figure 5.30

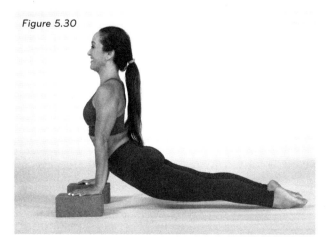

Figure 5.31

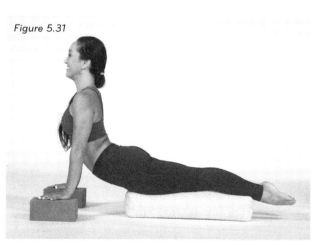

Sat (Six) Adho Mukha Svanasana (Downward-Facing Dog Pose)

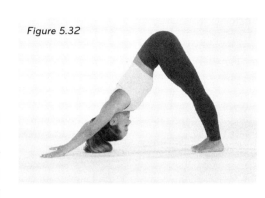

Figure 5.32

CHAIR VARIATION

Exhale and slide the chest back to Kumbhakasana, keeping the hands resting on the seat of the chair. Settle the soles of the feet down into the ground, and position the legs so the torso can relax down. Externally rotate the shoulders, and allow the chest and neck to drop down. Pivot at the hip joints and gaze toward the navel or the feet (see fig. 5.33). Stay for five breaths.

Exhale and slide the hands forward toward the front of the knees. Round the back and relax the neck. Maintain the activation of the pelvic floor. Gaze toward the navel (see fig. 5.34). Stay for five breaths. If this feels restrictive, try to relax the torso down on top of the thighs.

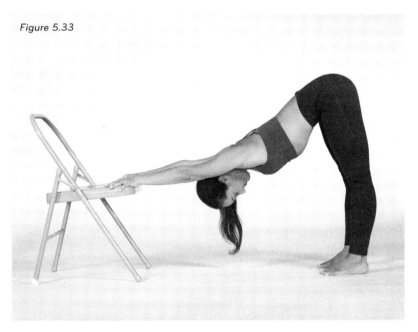

Figure 5.33

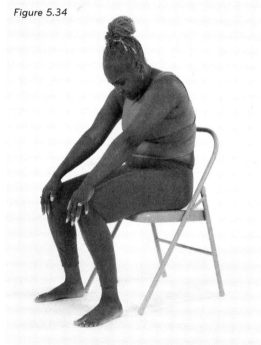

Figure 5.34

OTHER OPTIONS

Uttana Shishosana (Puppy Pose) is a great alternative to Adho Mukha Svanasana. There are many variations of this pose, just like there are many different types of puppies in the world. Be sure to find the one that best supports your practice. Enter this pose directly from whichever variation of Urdhva Mukha Svanasana works for you. Align the legs hip-width apart and the hands shoulder-width apart. Draw the muscles of the lower abdomen in toward the spine, and lift up along the center line with the pelvic floor. Externally rotate the shoulders and straighten the elbows. Rest the head on the floor. Stack the hips over the knees and allow the torso to

Figure 5.35

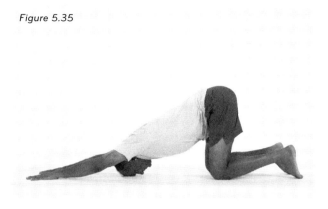

Figure 5.36

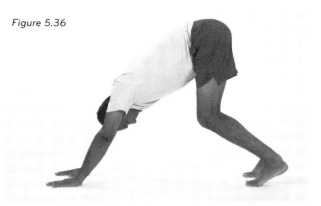

Figure 5.37

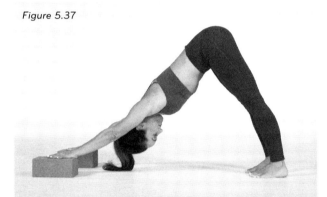

Figure 5.38

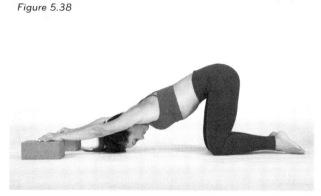

relax downward. Pivot at the hip joints to elongate the spine (see fig. 5.35). Maintain an active grounding through the legs, and either point or flex the feet. Stay for five breaths. Gaze toward the navel or the knees. Balasana (Child's Pose), with or without a bolster, is also a good alternative to Adho Mukha Svanasana.

Try bending the knees a bit in Adho Mukha Svanasana to distribute the weight more evenly throughout the body. Sometimes the weight tends to shift into the hands, and the back may round excessively. To work the key elements of the pose, try bending the knees and elevating the heels slightly to facilitate a deeper pivot at the hip joints (see fig. 5.36). Continuing on the blocks is also an option. Keep the hands centered on the two blocks, and inhale to send the hips back and up (see fig. 5.37), or sink the knees to come into Ardha Adho Mukha Svanasana (Half-Downward Dog) (see fig. 5.38).

SURYA NAMASKAR A

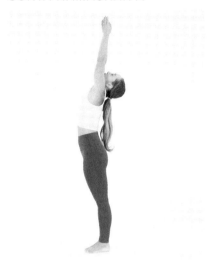

Ekam
Inhale

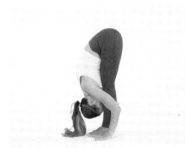

Dwe
Exhale

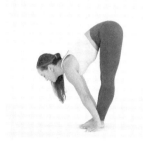

Trini
Inhale

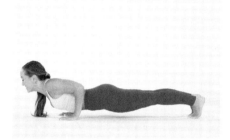

Chatuari—Chaturanga Dandasana
Exhale

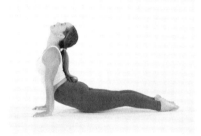

Panca—Urdhva Mukha Svanasana
Inhale

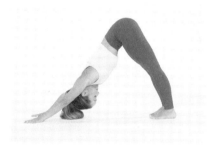

Sat—Adho Mukha Svanasana
Hold for five breaths

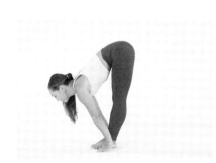

Sapta
Inhale

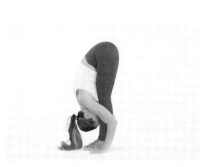

Astau
Exhale

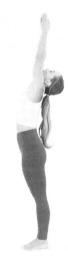

Nava
Inhale

Surya Namaskar B (Sun Salutation B)

Following the same flow of instructions as outlined for Surya Namaskar A, this second sequence of Sun Salutations adds two new poses to increase the cultivation of inner fire. Starting and ending in Utkatasana (Chair Pose) and adding in Virabhadrasana A (Warrior I) increases the cardio-vascular demand of the flow and helps warm up the body for practice. The basic flow of Surya Namaskar B is presented here, while the adaptations and variations of Utkatasana and Virabhadrasana A are outlined in chapter 7. The adaptations and variations for each of the other movements of Surya Namaskar B are the same as those recommended for Surya Namaskar A. While each of the movements outlined is traditionally said to be coordinated with one breath, feel free to take extra breaths to support the body's entry and exit from each of the movements. Coordinate each movement with either an inhalation or an exhalation, and continue to flow through the sequence in a safe manner for the body. Each movement in the sequence is held for one breath except for the last Adho Mukha Svanasana, which is held for five breaths. This entire sequence begins and ends in Samasthitih and is usually repeated three to five times.

SURYA NAMASKAR B

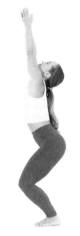

Ekam—Utkatasana
Inhale

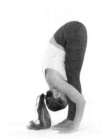

Dwe
Exhale

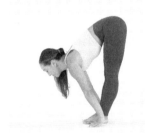

Trini
Inhale

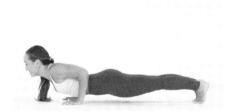

Chatuari—Chaturanga Dandasana
Exhale

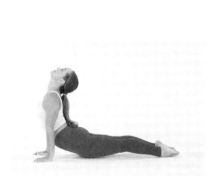

Panca—Urdhva Mukha Svanasana
Inhale

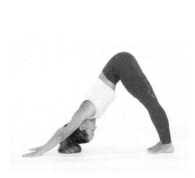

Sat—Adho Mukha Svanasana
Exhale

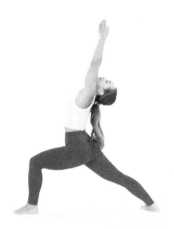

Sapta—Virabhadrasana A; right side
Inhale

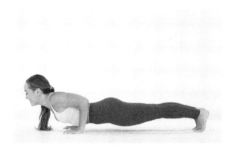

Astau—Chaturanga Dandasana
Exhale

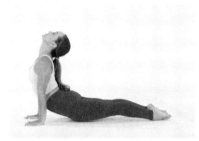

Nava—Urdhva Mukha Svanasana
Inhale

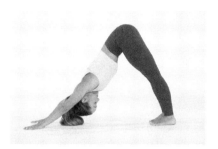

Dasa—Adho Mukha Svanasana
Exhale

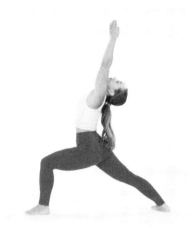

Ekadasa—Virabhadrasana A; left side
Inhale

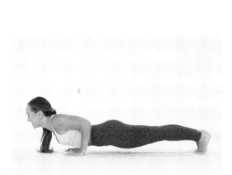

Dwadasa—Chaturanga Dandasana
Exhale

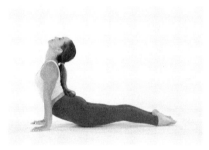

Trayodasa—Urdhva Mukha Svanasana
Inhale

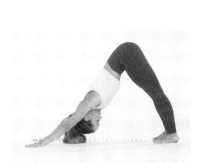

Chaturdasa—Adho Mukha Svanasana
Hold for five breaths

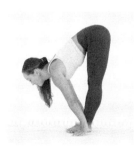

Sodasa
Inhale

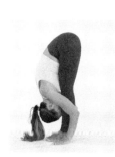

Saptadasa
Exhale

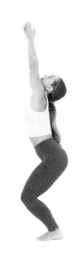

Astadasa—Utkatasana
Inhale

6

Standing Poses /
Foundational Asanas

THE STANDING POSES are considered the foundational asanas because the blueprint for every asana can be found within the architecture of this short series. By working dynamic flexibility, the body balances activation with release. The mind focuses and concentrates while working on coordinating breath with movement. Comprising a mixture of forward folds, external hip rotation, spinal twists, and more, there is a wide variety to explore within these asanas. Additionally, the pattern set by the student in this series of poses will lay the groundwork for movement mechanics in later, more complex asanas. Work subtly and with attention to detail, and do not force the body.

Padangusthasana (Big Toe Pose) and Padahastasana (Hands-to-Feet Pose)

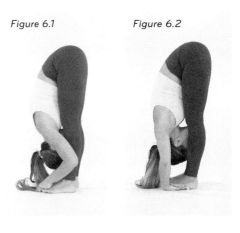

Figure 6.1   *Figure 6.2*

CHAIR VARIATION

Starting off in a seated position on a chair, align the feet to hip-width apart or slightly wider. Inhale as the spine lengthens and the muscles of the pelvic floor engage. Exhale as the torso pivots forward from the axis point of the hips. Reach down toward the feet and wrap the index fingers, middle fingers, and thumbs around the big toes. Keep the knees bent and the hips resting on the chair; inhale to create a bit more space between the ribs and the hips (see fig. 6.3). Exhale to fold the torso forward over the thighs, drop the head, gaze toward the nose, and settle into the pose for at least five deep breaths (see fig. 6.4).

Figure 6.3

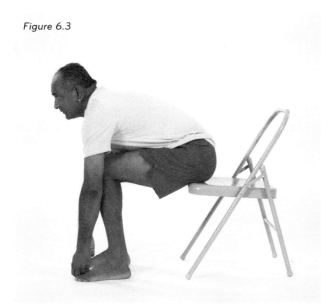

Figure 6.4

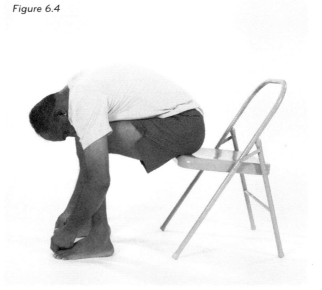

Continuing directly from Padangusthasana, inhale to lengthen the spine, shift the torso slightly away from the thighs, and place the hands as far under the soles of the feet as possible (see fig. 6.5). Look slightly up and forward, down the bridge of the nose. Exhale to fold forward and down. Maintain a conscious activation of the pelvic floor, and draw the muscles of the lower abdomen in to support the spine (see fig. 6.6). Relax the head, neck, and shoulders. Stay for at least five deep breaths. Inhale and lengthen the spine, shifting the gaze slightly forward and up. Exhale there to stabilize the pose. Inhale and return to a seated position on the chair.

Figure 6.5

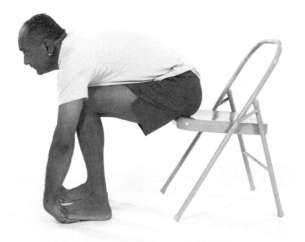

Figure 6.6

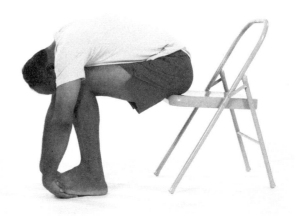

STANDING CHAIR VARIATION

Start off in a standing position in front of a chair, stepping the feet hip-width apart. Keeping the arms at the sides of the torso, inhale to create space, activate the muscles of the pelvic floor, and draw the muscles of the lower abdomen in toward the spine. Exhale and place the hands on the chair. Inhale again to draw the muscles of the abdomen even farther in toward the spine and maintain support from the pelvic floor (see fig. 6.7). Exhale to fold forward, relax the neck and shoulders, and pivot from the hips (see fig. 6.8). Stay for at least five breaths and repeat a second time.

Figure 6.7

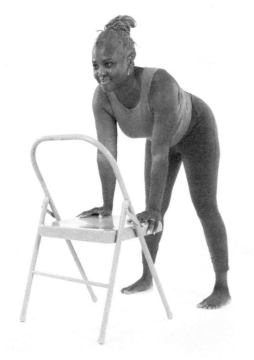

Figure 6.8

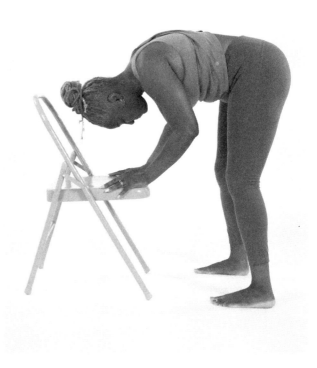

Figure 6.9

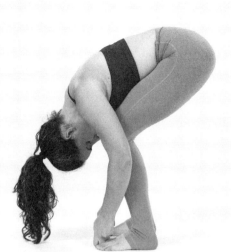

Figure 6.10

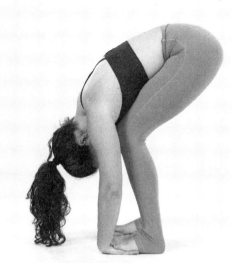

STANDING OPTION

Bending the knees is a good way to start working on forward folds. Start off in Samasthitih and step the feet hip-width apart. Keeping the arms at the sides of the torso, inhale to create space, activate the muscles of the pelvic floor, and draw the muscles of the lower abdomen in toward the spine. Exhale and bend the knees to fold forward and pivot at the hip joints. Wrap the thumbs, index fingers, and middle fingers around the big toes. Inhale again to create space by drawing the lower abdomen even farther in toward the spine. Exhale and fold forward to close the space between the torso and the thighs (see fig. 6.9). Stay for five breaths. Inhale again and lift the torso away from the thighs. Place the hands under the feet to prepare for Padahastasana. Maintaining the same muscular and internal activation, fold forward again (see fig. 6.10). Relax the neck and avoid pulling with the arms in either version of the forward fold. Gaze toward the nose. Stay for five breaths, then return to Samasthitih.

Figure 6.11

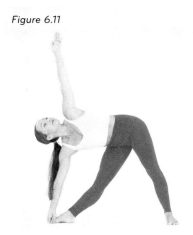

Utthita Trikonasana A (Extended Triangle Pose A)

CHAIR VARIATION

Start off in a standing position perpendicular to the chair. Inhale and step out to the right with the right leg, aligning the feet about three feet apart, adjusting for comfort and balance. Extend the arms outward in a T shape. Externally rotate the right hip joint and slightly turn the left hip inward to increase stability in the legs. Exhale as the torso folds lightly toward the right and descends gently toward the right hip crease (see fig. 6.12). Place the right hand on the seat of the chair and gaze up toward the left fingers or anyplace that feels comfortable. Stay for at least five breaths, then switch sides.

STANDING VARIATION

Starting off in Samasthitih, inhale and step out to the right with the right leg. Align the feet about three feet apart, adjusting for comfort and balance. Extend the arms outward in a T shape. Externally rotate the right hip joint and slightly turn the left hip inward to increase stability in the legs. Exhale as the torso folds lightly toward the right and descends gently toward the right hip crease (see fig. 6.13). Place the right hand on a block and gaze up toward the left fingers or anyplace that feels comfortable. Stay for at least five breaths, then switch sides.

Figure 6.12   Figure 6.13

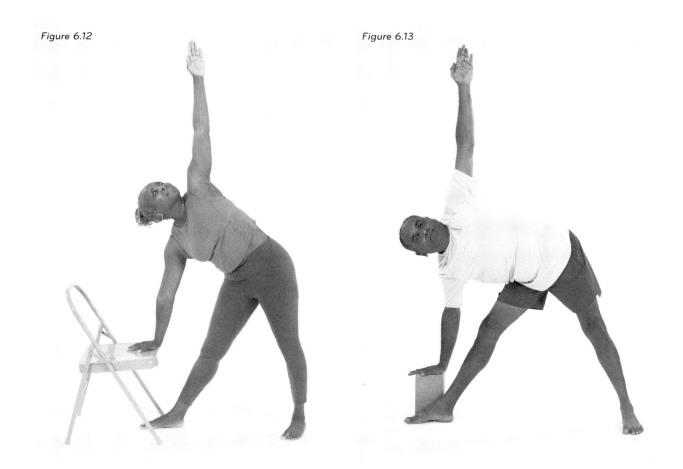

Utthita Trikonasana B (Extended Triangle Pose B)

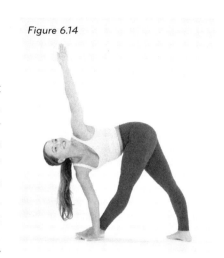

Figure 6.14

CHAIR VARIATION

Continuing directly from Trikonasana A on the left side, inhale and pivot the entire torso to face the chair. Align the hips to point directly forward. Externally rotate the left hip joint about forty-five degrees from the center line of the body. Keep the arms extended. Lead with the left hand as the torso folds slightly forward. Place the left hand firmly down on the chair aligned with either the left hip, the pubic bone, or the right hip. Twist the spine and lift the right arm overhead. Maintain spaciousness between the ribs and the hips (see fig. 6.15). Try different hand positions that best suit the body. If the forward fold begins to deepen, rest the forearm on the seat of the chair (see fig. 6.16). Avoid collapsing down. Lift the center of the chest, and reach out through the top of the head. Gaze up toward the left fingers or anyplace that feels comfortable. Stay for at least five deep breaths, then switch sides. Return to Samasthitih.

STANDING VARIATION

Continuing directly from Trikonasana A on the left side, inhale and lift the torso, extend the arms in a T shape, and stabilize the legs. Turn the pelvis toward the right, and maintain the same distance between the feet. Externally rotate the left hip joint forty-five degrees outward from the center line of the body. Reach forward with the left hand, and exhale as the left arm crosses the center line of the body and makes contact with a yoga block placed on the outer edge of the right foot. Root firmly down into the block with the strength of the arms and shoulders. Maintain spaciousness between the ribs and the hips (see fig. 6.17). Avoid collapsing down. Try different placements of the block to better support the body. Lift the center of the chest, and reach out through the top of the head. Gaze up toward the right fingers or anyplace that feels comfortable. Stay for at least five deep breaths, then switch sides. Return to Samasthitih.

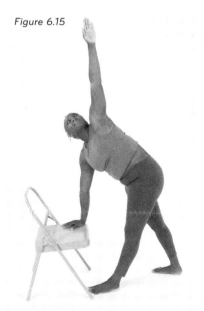

Figure 6.15

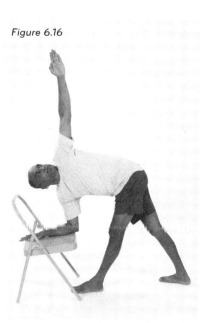

Figure 6.16

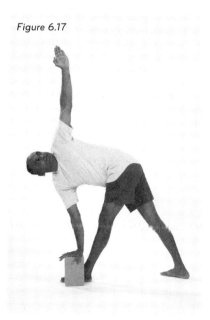

Figure 6.17

Figure 6.18

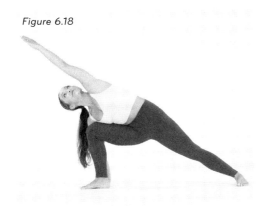

Utthita Parsvakonasana A
(Extended Side Angle Pose A)

CHAIR VARIATION

Start off seated on the chair with the feet hip-width apart; inhale as the legs move away from each other and the knees point in opposite directions. Turn the left hip slightly inward, straighten the left leg, and root down through the sole of the left foot. Rotate the right hip joint outward. Create space between the ribs and the hips. Draw the muscles of the lower abdomen in toward the spine, and activate the muscles of the pelvic floor. Exhale as the torso slides gently in toward the right hip crease. Bend the right elbow, stabilize the shoulder, and settle the right forearm on the right thigh toward the knee. Extend the left arm in line with the left side of the body, straighten the left arm, and externally rotate the left shoulder (see fig. 6.19). If both feet do not comfortably reach the floor, use a block to support the right foot or try a smaller chair (see fig. 6.20). Gaze up toward the left fingers. Hold the pose for at least five breaths, then switch sides.

Figure 6.19   *Figure 6.20*

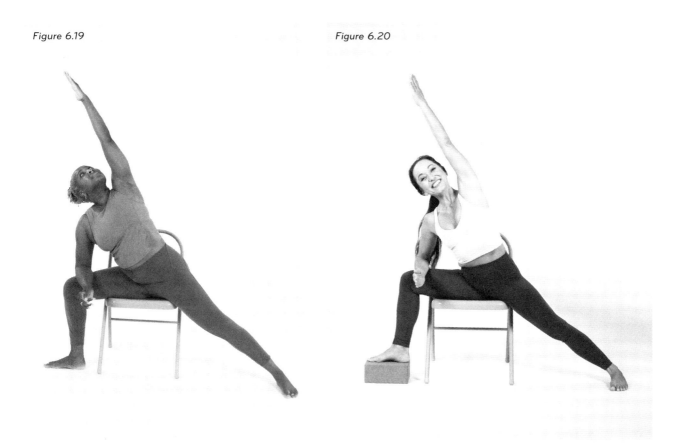

STANDING VARIATION

Start off in Samasthitih with the feet perpendicular to the chair; step out to the right side. Rotate the right hip externally, and turn the left hip slightly inward. Place the right foot slightly under the seat of the chair. Bend the right arm down toward the right ankle. Create space between the ribs and the hips. Draw the muscles of the lower abdomen in toward the spine, and activate the muscles of the pelvic floor. Exhale as the torso slides gently in toward the right hip crease. Bend the right elbow, stabilize the shoulder, and settle the right forearm on the seat of the chair (see fig. 6.21). Extend the left arm up in line with the left side of the body, straighten the left arm, and externally rotate the left shoulder. Try resting the right forearm on the right thigh (see fig. 6.22). Press actively down with the right arm, and lift the torso away to spiral the chest open and up. A block is a good intermediary step between the chair and the floor. Align the block with the right foot and root the right hand down on the block. Gaze up toward the left fingers. Hold the pose for at least five breaths, then switch sides.

Figure 6.21

Figure 6.22

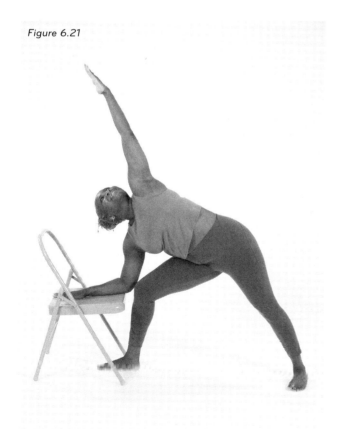

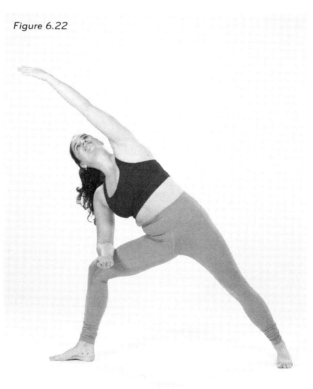

Figure 6.23

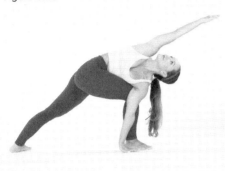

Utthita Parsvakonasana B
(Extended Side Angle Pose B)

CHAIR VARIATION

Continuing directly from Parsvakonasana A on the left side, bend the right knee, straighten the left leg, and lift the left heel off the ground. Inhale to lengthen the spine, lift the ribs away from the hips, maintain the activation of the pelvic floor, and draw the muscles of the lower abdomen in toward the spine. Exhale while gently clasping the backrest of the chair; twist the spine and gaze toward the right (see fig. 6.24). Think about each joint of the spine pivoting around the central axis. Be careful not to yank on the backrest to force the twist. Instead, focus on the inner sensation of twisting and lifting.

Another option is to slide the hips forward on the seat of the chair and pivot around so the left leg extends back and the right leg is supported by the chair. If the right foot does not comfortably reach the floor, use a block to provide a foundation for it. Exhale while gently twisting the torso to the right. Inhale and lengthen the torso away from the hips, twist around the central axis of the body and extend the arms (see fig. 6.25). If this feels comfortable, exhale and place the hands in prayer position. Gaze slightly to the right (see fig. 6.26). Stay for five breaths, then switch sides. Return to a comfortable seated position on the chair.

Extending the legs and twisting can be challenging and tricky, so if neither of these options work, feel free to explore what works for the body. Another variation could be to stack the legs hip-width apart, place a block on the thighs, root the right elbow down on the block, and twist the torso (see fig. 6.27). Continue to explore how best to work the fundamentals of this pose to best support the body.

Figure 6.24

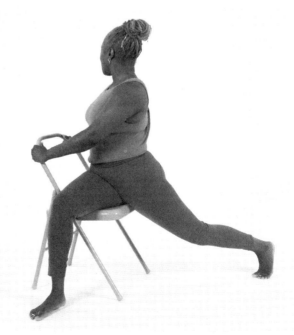

Figure 6.25

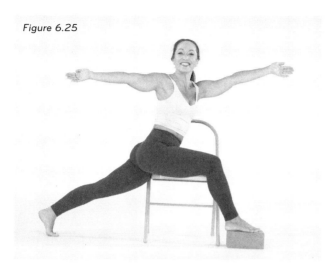

Figure 6.26

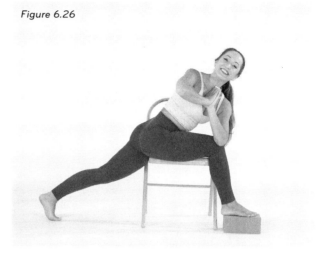

Figure 6.27

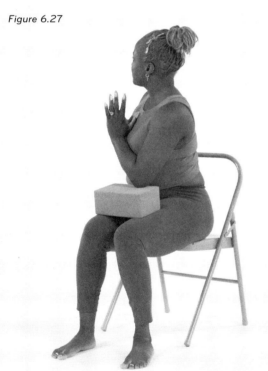

Figure 6.28

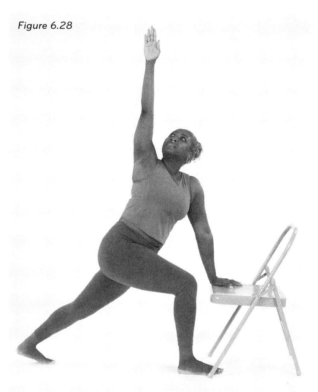

STANDING VARIATION

Continuing directly from Parsvakonasana A, pivot the entire body to the right, lift the left heel off the ground, and bend the right knee down over the ankle. Inhale to lengthen the spine, lift the ribs away from the hips, maintain the activation of the pelvic floor, and draw the muscles of the lower abdomen in toward the spine. Align the body in front of a chair or stable surface. Exhale while reaching the left hand down to the seat of the chair, twist the spine, and lift the right arm overhead using external rotation (see fig. 6.28).

If this feels comfortable, explore lowering the left hand. Instead of placing it on the seat of the chair, try placing it on the floor on the inside edge of the right foot. Align the left fingertips with the right toes, stabilize the shoulders, engage the pelvic floor, straighten the left leg, and gaze up toward the right fingertips (see figs. 6.29 and 6.30). The open-twist adaptation is especially useful for pregnant people; those with hip, shoulder, or spinal injuries; and bigger bodies.

Explore folding the torso around the thigh as another option to work this pose. Maintain a parallel position of the hips, and separate the feet by at least the length of one leg (between three and four feet). Sink the left knee toward the ground. If there is any discomfort in the knee, place a blanket or cushion under the knee. Align the right knee over the right ankle. If the knee is too far back, this will inhibit the twist; if the knee is too far forward, this will put too much pressure on the knee, ankle, and hips. Find the sweet spot around the vicinity of the ankle. Inhale and lengthen the spine, lift the ribs away from the hips, maintain the activation of the pelvic floor, and draw the muscles of the lower abdomen in toward the spine. Exhale and fold the torso around the outer edge of the right thigh. Drop the left shoulder as far down toward the right knee as possible. Draw the lower ribs in, and rotate each vertebra around the spinal axis. A gentle discomfort around the abdominal organs is to be expected here. Place the hands in prayer position, and firm the shoulder girdle (see fig. 6.31).

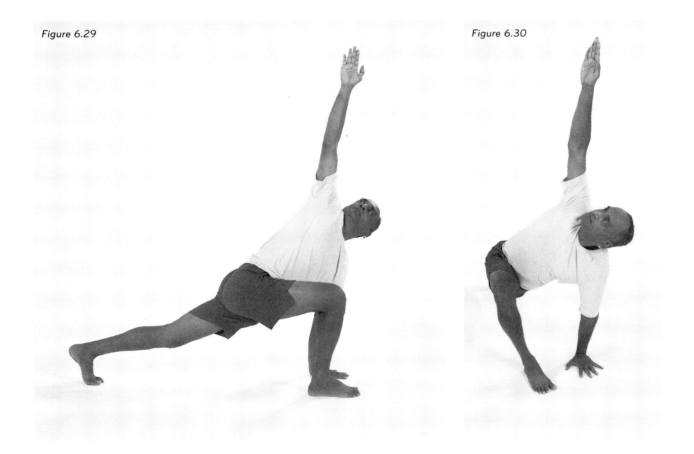

Figure 6.29

Figure 6.30

If this feels comfortable, try challenging the sense of balance. Increase the muscular activation of the legs, torso, and pelvic floor. Maintain a firm gaze on a single point over the right shoulder. Inhale and send the right knee slightly forward; straighten the left leg completely to come into a lifted lunge (see fig. 6.32). While balance is challenged with the back heel off the ground, the parallel position makes the twisting action more accessible. If the twist feels comfortable, and the torso slides down around the outer edge of the right knee, try placing the left heel on the floor. Externally rotate the left hip joint about forty-five degrees and allow the right heel to extend toward the floor (see fig. 6.34). Stabilize the left leg by activating the quadriceps. Keep sending the right knee forward over the right ankle. Avoid hiking one hip up to plant the back leg. Keep the pelvis level. While this sequence is presented progressively, it may be appropriate to choose one option from this sequence that best supports the practice. Each variation can be entered directly, or the entire sequence can be practiced daily to deepen the twisting work. Gaze over the right shoulder. Stay for five breaths, then switch sides. Return to Samasthitih.

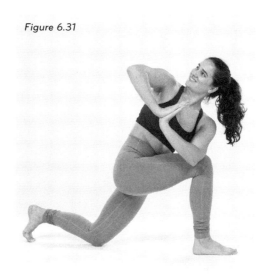

Figure 6.31

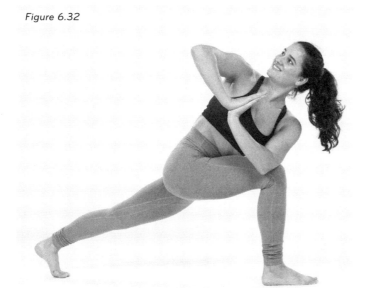

Figure 6.32

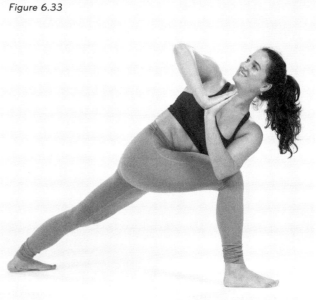

Figure 6.33

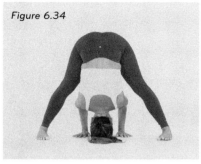

Figure 6.34

Prasarita Padottanasana A, B, C, and D (Wide-Legged Forward Bend A, B, C, and D)

CHAIR VARIATION

Start off in Samasthitih facing the chair. Inhale and step the right foot out to the right. Align the feet four to five feet apart. Activate the muscles of the pelvic floor, lift the ribs away from the hips, draw the muscles of the lower abdomen in toward the spine, and firm the quadriceps. Exhale and place the forearms on the chair; pivot forward from the hip joints, looking up to prepare (see fig. 6.38). Exhale, drop the head down, and settle into the pose for five deep breaths (see fig. 6.39). Inhale, return to the preparation step (see fig. 6.40), and exhale. Inhale to come all the way back to standing. Repeat the same variation for Prasarita Padottanasana B and D.

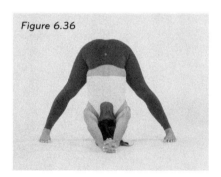

Figure 6.35

Figure 6.38

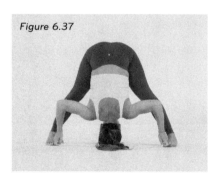

Figure 6.36

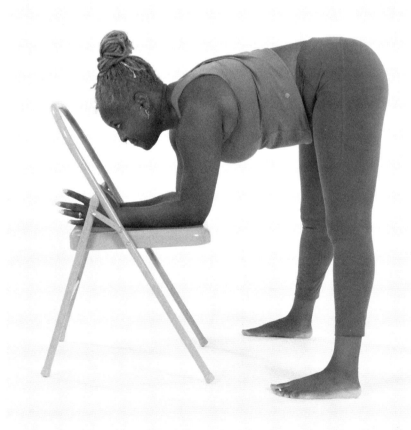

Figure 6.37

Figure 6.39

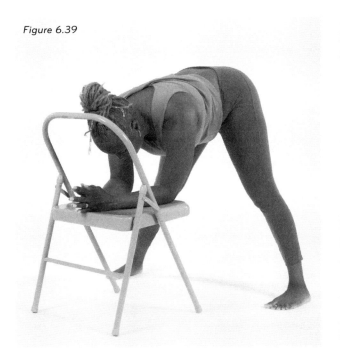

Figure 6.40

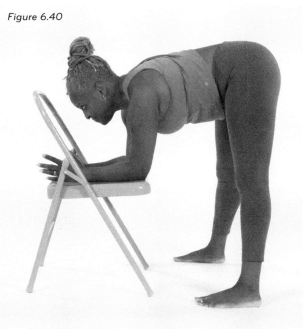

WALL VARIATION

For Prasarita Padottanasana C, use the wall to support the back. Face the wall and leave about one foot between the feet and the wall. Inhale and engage the muscles of the pelvic floor; lift the ribs away from the hips. Exhale, pivot forward into the hip joints to fold forward, and place the back against the wall. Extend the arms up the wall and internally rotate the shoulders (see fig. 6.41). Gaze toward the nose. Stay for five breaths, then return to standing. If the wall support feels comfortable, explore all four poses in this sequence with the same wall support.

Figure 6.41

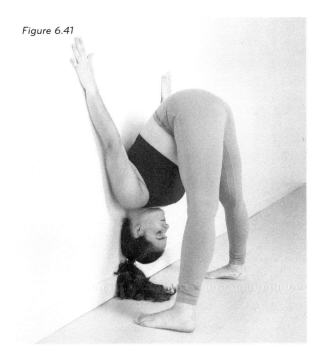

Figure 6.42

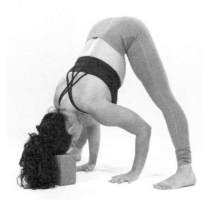

BLOCK VARIATION

Try using a block to support the head and bring the floor closer. Having support under the head lessens the pressure on the hamstrings, alleviates fear, and allows the body to relax. Place the block six inches to one foot in front of the feet, and align it with the center of the torso. Inhale and engage the muscles of the pelvic floor; lift the ribs away from the hips. Exhale, pivot forward into the hip joints to fold forward, and place the head on the block. All four variations of this pose sequence can be practiced with the block support under the head. After each variation, inhale to come back to standing and fold forward again (see figs. 6.42 and 6.43).

For the Prasarita Padottanasana C variation, explore holding a strap to give the shoulders more space. Prepare by holding a strap behind the back from standing. Internally rotate the shoulders, holding the strap firmly. Maintain the grip and the rotation of the shoulders while folding forward. This can be practiced with or without the block to support the head (see fig. 6.44).

Figure 6.43

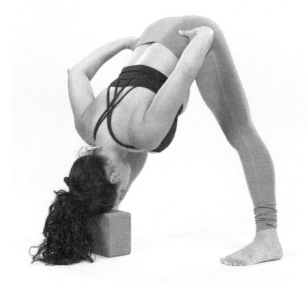

Figure 6.44

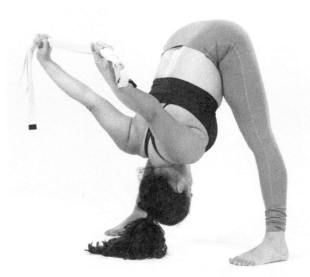

Parsvottanasana (Pyramid Pose)

Figure 6.45

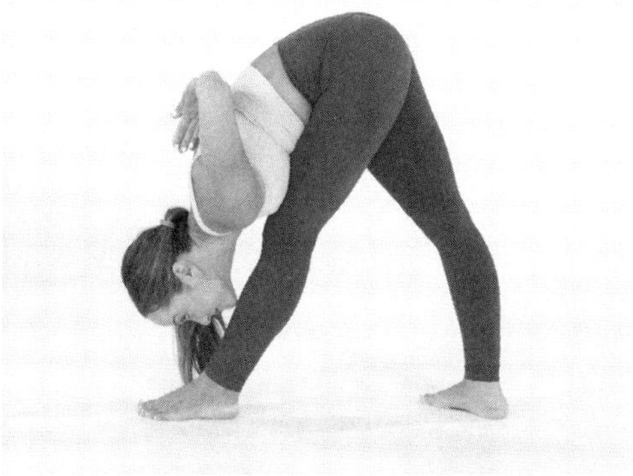

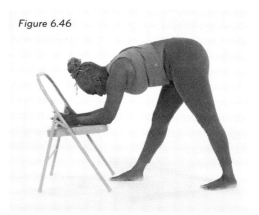

CHAIR VARIATION

Start off in Samasthitih. Inhale and step the right foot out to the right. Place the chair at the back of the mat with the seat of the chair facing toward the front of the mat. Align the torso facing the chair and keep the feet two to three feet apart. Rotate the left foot approximately forty-five degrees or less out to the side. Exhale while folding forward, rest the forearms on the chair, and relax the head down (see fig. 6.46). Stay here for five breaths, then switch sides. Return to Samasthitih.

STANDING VARIATION

Figure 6.46

Start off in Samasthitih. Step the feet out to three feet or less apart. Turn the right foot out to forty-five degrees, and turn the hips and whole body to face the right foot. Externally rotate the left hip joint to forty-five degrees or more. Place a block in the highest position on each side of the right foot. Align the feet so that the heels track along the center line of the mat or so that the heels track with just a bit of space around the center line of the mat, whichever best supports the pelvis. Inhale to lengthen the spine, activate the pelvic floor, and draw the muscles of the lower abdomen in toward the spine. Activate the quadriceps and the muscles of the legs to support the pose. Exhale and pivot forward into the hip joints, placing the hands on the blocks (see fig. 6.47). Gaze forward toward the right toes. Stay for five breaths, then pivot and repeat on the other side.

Once the legs and hips feel strong enough and the forward fold feels accessible, explore lifting the hands off the blocks. Internally rotate the shoulders and gently reach the hands around the back to hold the elbows with the opposite hands (see fig. 6.48). Gaze forward toward the right toes. Stay for five breaths, then pivot and repeat on the other side.

Figure 6.47

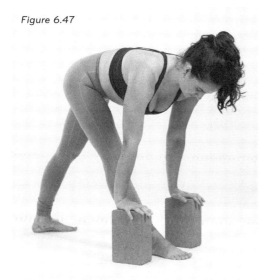

Figure 6.48

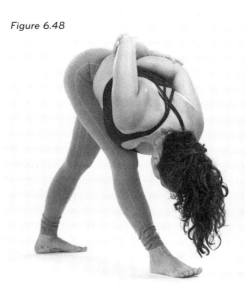

7

Primary Series

THERE ARE SIX SERIES in the Ashtanga Yoga method, and the Primary Series is considered the basis from which the entire practice unfolds. Called Yoga Chikitsa in Sanskrit, the Primary Series of Ashtanga Yoga establishes a level of health, strength, and flexibility in the body and mind and prepares the nervous system for deeper states of meditation and reflection. It has been more commonly accepted to adapt and adjust the asanas of the Primary Series in group classes. Many accessible variations of these asanas are already familiar. When working with the adaptations of the asanas, remember to reflect on what the essence of each asana is for you and find the work that best supports your body and mind.

Utthita Hasta Padangusthasana
(Extended Hand-to-Big-Toe Pose)

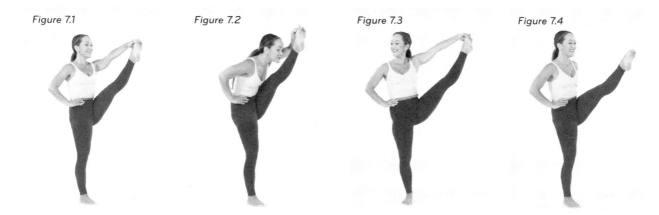

Figure 7.1   Figure 7.2   Figure 7.3   Figure 7.4

CHAIR VARIATION

Start off in a seated position on the chair. Keep the left foot on the floor; wrap a strap around the right foot, and hold on to the strap with both hands. Bend the right knee if necessary to place the strap comfortably. Inhale to straighten and lift the leg (see fig. 7.5). Stay for five breaths. Align the right leg with the right hip joint, keeping the torso upright. Gaze toward the right toes. Exhale and switch both sides of the strap to the right hand, rotate the right hip joint externally and guide the right leg out to the side (see fig. 7.6). Gaze toward the left. Stay for five breaths. Inhale and bring the right leg back to a parallel position in front; release the strap, place both hands on the waist, and keep the right leg elevated (see fig. 7.7). Gaze toward the right toes. Stay for five breaths.

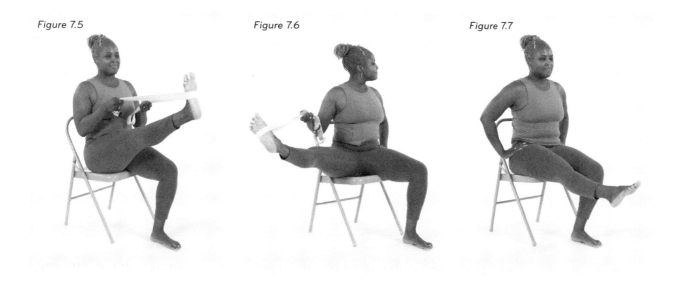

Figure 7.5   Figure 7.6   Figure 7.7

Figure 7.8

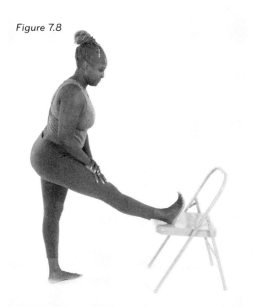

For another option, start off in Samasthitih facing the chair. Inhale and bend the right knee to place the right foot on the seat of the chair. Straighten the right leg and place both hands on the right thigh (see fig. 7.8), Gaze toward the right toes or anywhere that feels comfortable. Stay for five breaths. Inhale, lift the right foot off the chair, and return to standing. Pivot the entire body to the left, away from the chair. Externally rotate the right hip joint, and turn the right leg outward. Inhale and bend the right knee, and place the right foot on the chair, maintaining the external rotation of the right hip joint. Place the left hand on the waist and the right hand on the right thigh; gaze toward the left (see fig. 7.9). Stay for five breaths. Inhale, lift the right foot off the chair, and return to standing. Walk around to the back of the chair or find a slightly lower pedestal. Inhale, lift the right leg, and nestle the toes on the back bar of the chair (see fig. 7.10). Gaze toward the right toes or anywhere that feels comfortable. Stay for five breaths, then return to standing. Repeat on the left side.

Figure 7.9

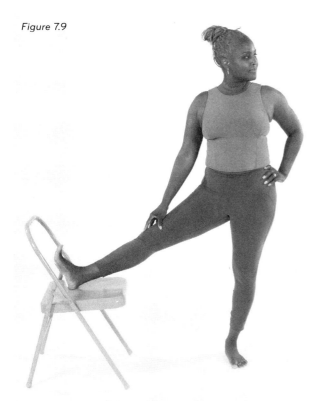

Figure 7.10

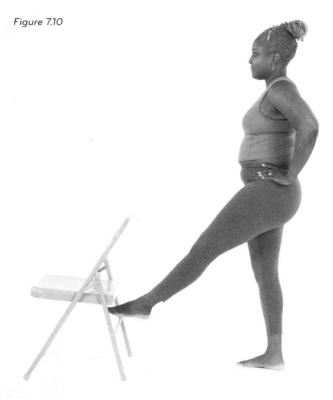

STANDING VARIATION

Start off in Samasthitih. Bend the right knee, and wrap a strap around the right foot. Hold both ends of the strap with the right hand. Inhale, lift the right leg and straighten as much as is comfortable. Place the left hand on the waist and gaze toward the right toes (see fig. 7.11). Stay for five breaths. Exhale and externally rotate the right hip joint to bring the right leg out to the side. Place the left hand on the waist and look toward the left (see fig. 7.12). Stay for five breaths. Inhale and bring the right leg back to center. Release the strap. Lift the right leg without the strap and keep it straight, even if the foot remains just a few inches off the ground. Gaze toward the right toes. Stay for five breaths, then repeat on the left side. Return to Samasthitih.

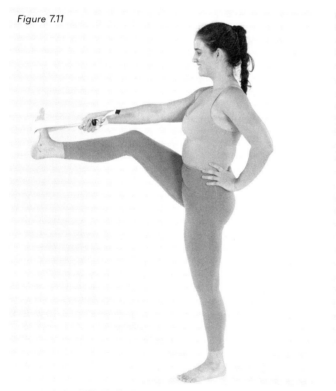

Figure 7.11

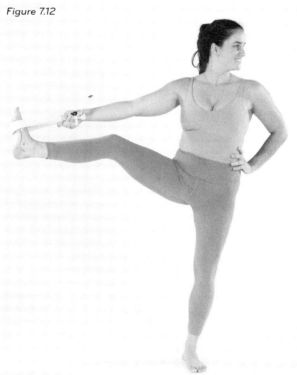

Figure 7.12

Figure 7.13

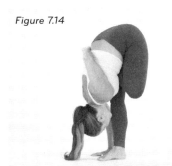

Figure 7.14

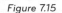

Ardha Baddha Padmottanasana
(Bound Lotus Forward Fold Pose)

CHAIR VARIATION

Stand next to the chair with the side of the left leg facing it. Place a block next to the left foot, hold on to the chair, and gently step the right foot onto the block. Externally rotate the right hip joint, lightly press the right heel toward the left lower leg or ankle, and ground through the ball of the right foot. Draw the right hand up to the center of the chest when balance feels established (see fig. 7.15). Gaze toward any single point ahead or slightly forward and down that helps with balance. Stay for five breaths, then repeat on the left side. Return to Samasthitih.

Try the pose without the block to challenge balance and flexibility. Stand behind the chair in Samasthitih, place the hands lightly on the backrest of the chair, and glide the right foot up along the left calf muscle by externally rotating the right hip joint. Stabilize with the muscles of the pelvic floor, activate the deep six hip rotator muscles around the right hip joint, lift up along the spinal axis, and root down through the left leg (see fig. 7.16). Gaze toward any single point ahead or slightly forward and down that helps with balance. Stay for five breaths, then repeat on the left side. Return to Samasthitih.

Figure 7.15

Figure 7.16

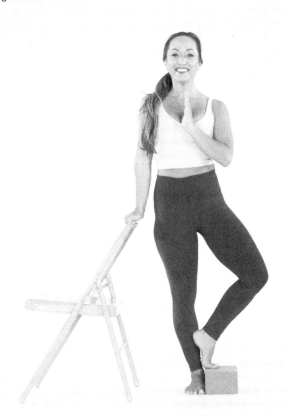

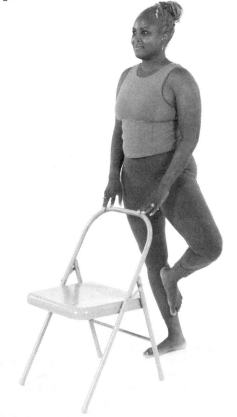

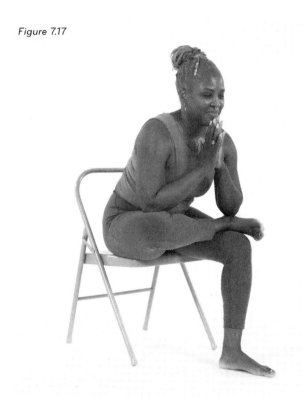

Figure 7.17

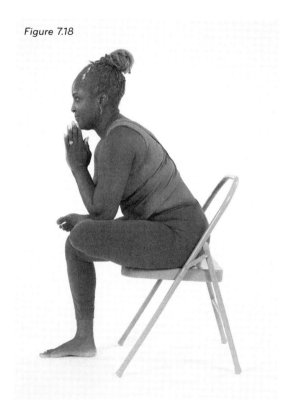

Figure 7.18

Try Eka Pada Utkatasana (Figure Four or One-Footed Chair Pose) on a chair or a variation of seated Kapotasana (Pigeon Pose) for maximum stability. Starting off in a seated position on the chair, slide the buttocks slightly forward. Ground through the left leg, externally rotate the right hip joint, and place the right foot on the lower part of the left thigh (toward the knee) to make a number 4 shape with the legs. Tilt the pelvis anteriorly a few degrees, close the hip creases, draw the muscles of the lower abdomen in toward the spine, and lean forward a little. Do not overly round the spine. Instead, relax the back muscles, elongate the spine, and use the hip joints as a fulcrum point for movement. Rest the elbows on the upper inner edge of the right thigh and the outer inner edge of the right foot (figs. 7.17 and 7.18). Gaze toward any single point slightly forward and down that helps with balance. Stay for five breaths, then repeat on the left side. Return to Samasthitih.

STANDING VARIATION

Start off in Samasthitih with the bases of the big toes aligned. If balance feels well established, then try this on the mat in the middle of the room. Bend the left knee slightly, externally rotate the right hip joint, point the right knee out to the side, draw the right foot up along the front of the left leg to make a number four shape with the legs. If the right leg feels comfortably situated, draw the hands into prayer position (see fig. 7.19). Gaze toward any single point ahead or slightly forward and down that helps with balance. Stay for five breaths, then repeat on the left side. Return to Samasthitih.

Figure 7.19   *Figure 7.20*   *Figure 7.21*

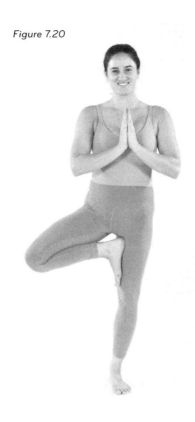

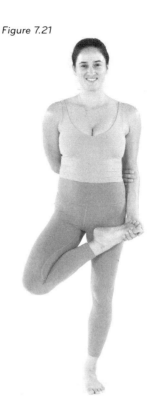

Try the same pose with a closed knee. Start off in Samasthitih with the bases of the big toes aligned. Externally rotate the right hip joint, and draw the right foot up along the inner edge of the left leg with the hands. Snuggle the right heel as high as possible along the left inner thigh. Avoid pressing the right foot into the left knee—place it either above or below the knee. Once the right foot is firmly positioned, draw the hands to prayer position at the center of the chest. Stabilize with the muscles of the pelvic floor, activate the deep six hip rotator muscles around the right hip joint, lift up along the spinal axis, and root down through the left leg (see fig. 7.20). This asana is often referred to as Vrksasana (Tree Pose). Gaze toward any single point ahead or slightly forward and down that helps with balance. Stay for five breaths, then repeat on the left side. Return to Samasthitih.

Now try a standing Ardha Padmasana (Half-Lotus Pose). Continuing directly from the preceding variation of Vrksasana, reach down with both hands, extend the right ankle, and clasp the right foot. Slide the right foot up toward the left hip crease, keeping a gentle activation in the right foot and ankle. Check the right knee to be sure there is no pressure or pain, and only proceed once the right knee is safe. Once the right foot and knee are comfortably stable in the pose, release the grip with the right hand. Slide the right hand around the back, and hold the left elbow; continue holding on to the right foot with the left hand (see fig. 7.21). Gaze toward any single point ahead or slightly forward and down that helps with balance. Stay for five breaths, then repeat on the left side. Return to Samasthitih.

Utkatasana (Chair Pose)

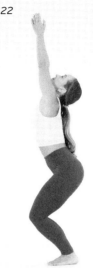

Figure 7.22

CHAIR VARIATION

Start off seated on the chair and slide the hips forward to the front of the chair. Align the feet either hip-width apart or together, depending on what feels more stable. Firmly press the feet down, and be sure the hips are far enough forward to ground through the feet. Activate the leg muscles, the pelvic floor, and the muscles of the lower abdomen. Inhale as the spine lengthens, the shoulders rotate externally, and the arms lift. Keep the arms shoulder-width apart, and gaze forward. Pivot the torso slightly into the hips to deepen the hip creases (see fig. 7.23). It should feel as though the body is just about to stand up from the chair. Stay for five breaths, then sit back in the chair.

OTHER OPTIONS

Try practicing Utkatasana with a block between the knees. The added space may help the hips bend more deeply and prevent stress on the front of the hip joints. Align the feet hip-width apart and place a block between the knees. Actively squeeze the block with the full strength of the legs. Inhale and extend the arms, lift the ribs away from the hips, externally rotate the shoulders, and reach up with the sternum. Gaze forward.

Figure 7.23

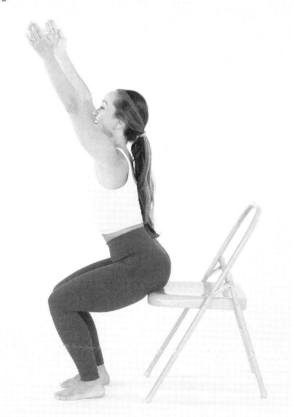

Figure 7.24

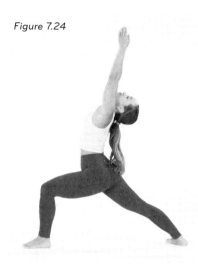

Virabhadrasana A (Warrior I)

CHAIR VARIATION

Start off seated on the chair, and slide the hips forward to the front of the chair. Turn the entire body to the right and check to see if the feet comfortably rest on the floor. If the feet are not firmly planted on the floor, place a block on the right side of and perpendicular to the chair. Place the right foot on the block and circle the left leg around to the other side of the chair. Externally rotate the left hip joint, and turn the left foot out about forty-five degrees. Keep the pelvis and torso oriented toward the right foot. Inhale as the spine lengthens along the central axis, the ribs lift away from the hips, and the shoulders rotate externally as they float up (see fig. 7.25). Activate the leg muscles, the pelvic floor, the muscles of the lower abdomen, and the spinal extensors. Think about lifting the body off the chair with the strength of the legs and the pelvic floor. Gaze forward. Stay for five breaths, then switch sides.

Figure 7.25

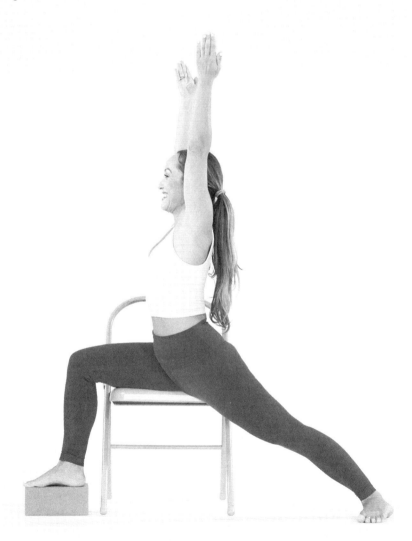

OTHER OPTIONS

Extending the arms directly above the head, placing the palms together, and looking up can be challenging if the shoulders and neck are tight or sore. Step forward with the right foot, externally rotate the left hip joint and lift the torso. Inhale and bring the hands together in prayer position (see fig. 7.26). Externally rotate the shoulders, lift the arms, align the hands as close to above the shoulders and along the center line as possible. Lift the ribs away from the hips, and root down into the ground with the strength of the legs (see fig. 7.27). Engage the pelvic floor, and draw the muscles of the lower abdomen in toward the spine. Gaze forward. Do not attempt to bring the hands toward each other or look up until the shoulders and upper back feel comfortable in the extended position. Explore how much distance between the legs feels best for the body. A narrow stance may feel safer in regard to balance. A wider stance may help access more flexibility but can challenge balance. Bending the knee too deeply may strain the joint, but bending the knee over the ankle of the forward leg may help strengthen the leg. Try different options and find what works best. Stay for five breaths, then switch sides.

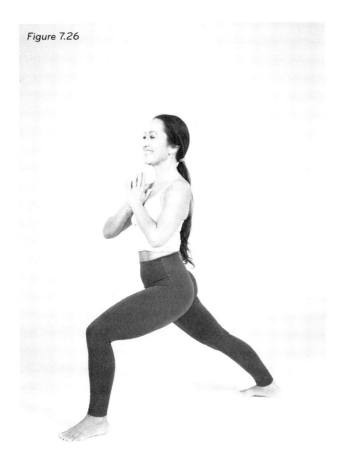

Figure 7.26

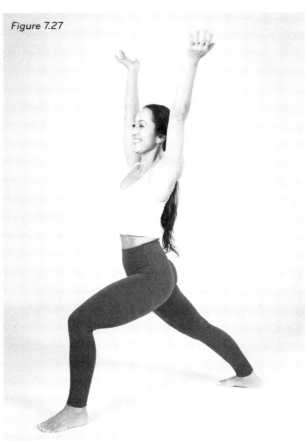

Figure 7.27

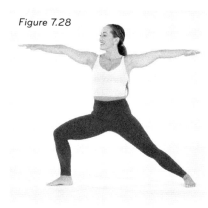

Figure 7.28

Virabhadrasana B (Warrior II)

CHAIR VARIATION

Continuing directly from Virabhadrasana A from the Chair Variation, stay on the left side. Continue grounding through the legs and feet, open the pelvis so the orientation of the pubic bone and torso falls in the midline between the knees. Extend the arms out to a T shape, separate the shoulder blades while keeping them down the back, maintain the space between the ribs and the hips, and gaze toward the left fingers (see fig. 7.29). Think about lifting the body off the chair with the strength of the legs and the pelvic floor. If the block is not necessary to ground the foot, then try the pose without it (see fig. 7.30). Stay for five breaths, then repeat on the other side. Sit back in the chair.

Figure 7.29

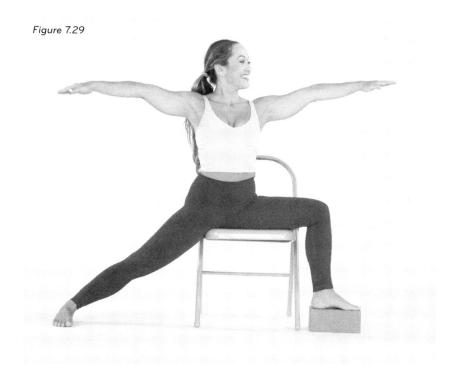

Figure 7.30

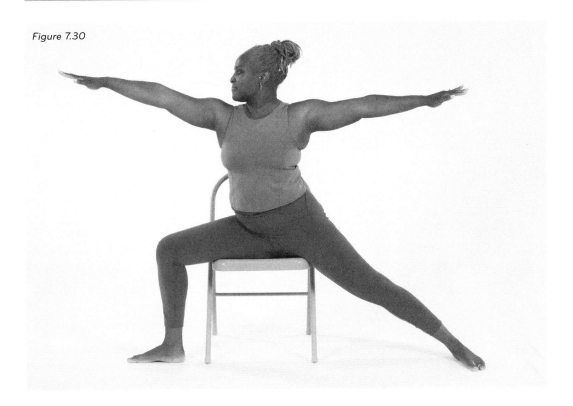

OTHER OPTIONS

To work on balance, try this pose from standing. Continuing from Virabha-drasana A, use the chair for support. Stand behind the chair and clasp the back. Turn the pelvis toward the chair so the orientation of the pubic bone and torso falls in the midline between the knees. Gaze forward and main-tain contact with the back of the chair (see fig. 7.31). Stay for five breaths, then switch sides.

Figure 7.31

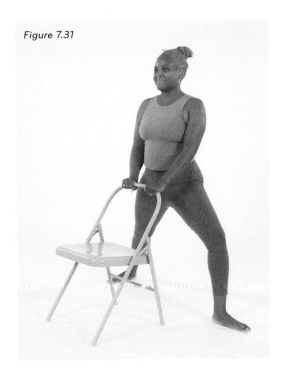

Figure 7.32

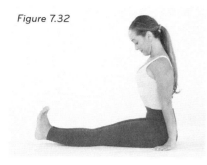

Figure 7.33

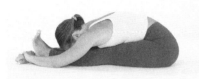

Dandasana (Staff Pose)/Paschimottanasana (Westward-Facing Stretch/Seated Forward Bend)

CHAIR VARIATION

Start off seated on the chair. Stay seated for five breaths to stabilize and center the body and mind. Place a block or footrest in front of the chair at about the length of the legs. Pivot forward toward the front of the chair and place both feet on the block. Wrap a strap around both feet, and gently engage the shoulders to support the torso. Engage the muscles of the quadriceps. Inhale and engage the muscles of the pelvic floor, lift the ribs away from the hips, draw the muscles of the lower abdomen in toward the spine, and pivot forward at the hip joints (see fig. 7.34). Stay for five breaths. Inhale to lengthen the spine, then exhale to fold forward again. Stay for an additional five breaths. Gaze toward the nose or the toes.

FLOOR VARIATION

Sit on a folded blanket or towel to elevate the hips and encourage a gentle rotation of the pelvis toward an anterior tilt. Situate the sitting bones at the middle to back of the blanket, bend the knees slightly, and wrap a strap around the middle of the soles of the feet. Extend the legs as much as feels comfortable. Inhale to prepare as the spine lengthens, the pelvic floor activates, and the quadriceps engage. Exhale as the shoulder blades draw down, the back muscles elongate and relax, and the torso pivots forward at the hip joints (see fig. 7.35). Gaze toward the toes. Stay for five breaths, then relax and repeat one more time. Be careful not to use the strap like a rope and pull on it. Instead, focus on the internal work of the forward fold.

Note that if the entire practice is to be done on a chair, it is always possible to repeat the Chair Variation provided for Padangusthasana and Padahastasana for this pose.

Figure 7.34

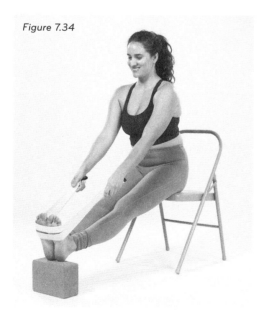

Figure 7.35

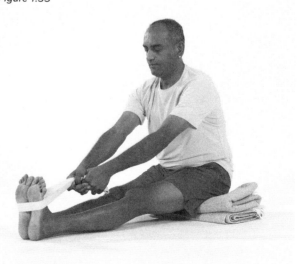

Purvottanasana (Eastward-Facing Stretch Plank Pose)

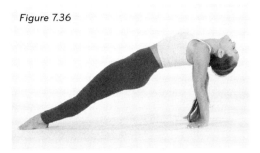

Figure 7.36

CHAIR VARIATION

Start off seated on the chair; slide the hips forward to the very front of the chair. Bend the knees and the elbows. Place the hands on the back of the seat, with the fingers pointing toward the front of the chair. Exhale as the hips slide slightly off the chair and dip down. Inhale as the hips lift, the arms straighten, the back muscles activate, and the legs and pelvic floor engage to support the spine. Keep the muscles of the lower abdomen drawn in, and breathe into the chest to lift the ribs away from the hips (see fig. 7.37). Look up. Stay for five breaths, then return to seated.

Figure 7.37

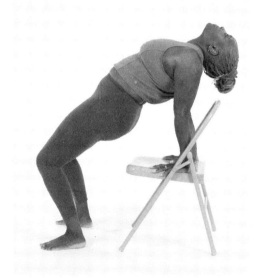

   Here is another option. Stand about one foot in front of the chair, bend the knees and elbows, and place the hands on the front of the seat of the chair. Hold on to the front corners of the seat, and turn the fingers slightly forward. Exhale as the hips dip down. Inhale and lift the hips, straighten the legs and arms, activate the back and legs, and engage the pelvic floor to support the spine. Keep the muscles of the lower abdomen drawn in, and breathe into the chest to lift the ribs away from the hips (see fig. 7.37). Look either at the nose or gently up. Stay for five breaths, then return to seated or standing.

FLOOR VARIATION

Start off seated on the floor. Place the legs slightly wider than hip-width apart and the feet slightly forward of the pelvis. Place the hands at least one foot behind the hips. Point the fingers toward the hips. Inhale as the hips lift, the arms straighten, the back muscles activate, and the legs and pelvic floor engage to support the spine. Keep the muscles of the lower abdomen drawn in, and breathe into the chest to lift the ribs away from the hips (see fig. 7.38). Look at the nose. Stay for five breaths, then return to seated. If the legs feel unstable, it may be useful to place a block between the knees for added stability.

Figure 7.38

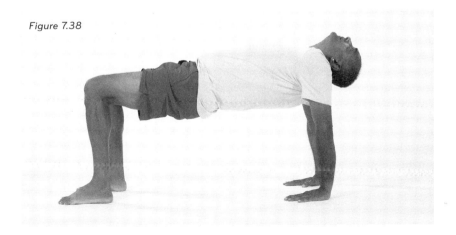

Figure 7.39

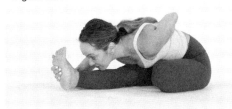

Ardha Baddha Padma Paschimottanasana (Half-Bound Lotus Forward Bend)

CHAIR VARIATION

Start off seated in a chair. Place a block on the floor a few feet in front of the chair, and place both feet on the block. Externally rotate the right hip joint, and slide the right foot up along the top of the left leg. Inhale and wrap a strap around the right foot; pass the right hand around the back and grasp the strap to help support the foot. Internally rotate the right shoulder, and align the torso forward toward the left leg. Keep the left leg engaged. Exhale and fold forward gently; reach the left hand down along the left thigh, and gaze toward the left toes or the nose (see fig. 7.40). Stay for five breaths, then repeat on the other side. Return to seated.

FLOOR VARIATION

Start off seated on the floor. Externally rotate the right hip joint. Place a block under the right knee to support it and prevent injury and stress. Stabilize the left leg, and firm the muscles of the left quadriceps. Place a strap around the right foot, and reach around the back with the right hand to grasp the strap. Internally rotate the right shoulder. Reach the left arm down along the shinbone to prepare for the forward fold. Inhale and lengthen the spine, lift the ribs away from the hips, activate the muscles of the pelvic floor, and draw the muscles of the lower abdomen in toward the spine. Exhale and pivot at the hip joints to fold forward (see fig. 7.41). Do not pull or force the body. Breathe deeply and focus on the subtlety of the inner sensations. Gaze toward the left toes. Stay for five breaths, then repeat on the other side. Return to seated.

Figure 7.40

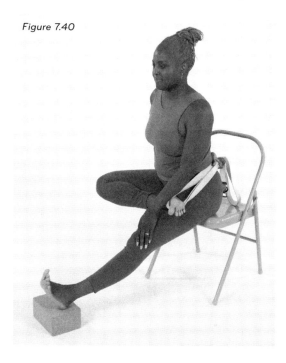

Figure 7.41

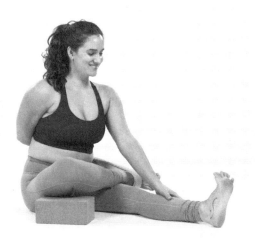

Tiryang Mukha Ekapada Paschimottanasana (Three-Limbed Forward Fold Pose)

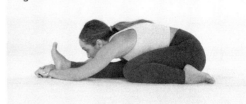

Figure 7.42

CHAIR VARIATION

Start off seated on a chair. Place a block on the floor in front of the chair about the distance of the leg. Rest the left heel firmly on the center of the block. Fold the right leg back, internally rotate the right hip joint, bend the right knee gently, extend the right ankle, and curl the right toes slightly. Allow the weight of the right leg to rest gently on the ball of the right foot. Place both hands on the left thigh and gaze toward the left toes (see fig. 7.43). Stay for five breaths, then repeat on the other side. Return to Dandasana.

If that option doesn't work well, try this one. Start off seated on a chair. Slide the hips forward to the front edge of the chair and hold on to the seat with both hands. Internally rotate the right hip joint and slide the right leg under the chair, aligning the leg toward the inside edge of the chair near the legs. Point the right foot as it extends back. Bend the left knee and plant the left foot firmly on the floor. Engage the quadriceps of the left leg, firm the muscles of the pelvic floor, maintain stability in the shoulder girdle, and lift the ribs away from the hips (see fig. 7.44). Gaze forward. Stay for five breaths, then repeat on the other side. Return to seated.

Figure 7.43

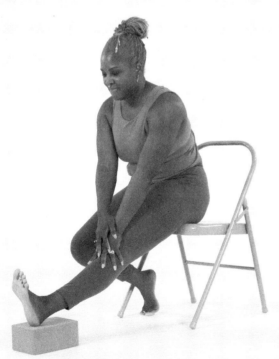

Figure 7.44

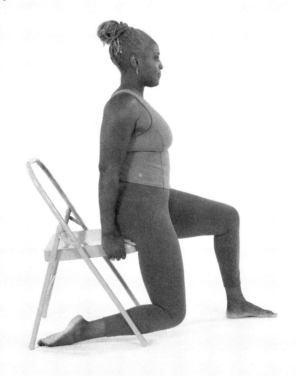

FLOOR VARIATION

Starting off in Dandasana, place a block under both sitting bones. Turn the block to the lowest position, and place the long edge parallel to the back of the mat. Once the pelvis is firmly supported by the block, internally rotate the right hip joint, fold the right knee back, curl the right toes under, and point the foot. Snuggle the foot in toward the outer edge of the right hip. Use a strap to lasso the left foot and align the center of the chest toward the left knee. Inhale to prepare, activate the pelvis floor, lift the ribs away from the hips, and create space along the front of the body. Exhale to enter the asana, gaze toward the toes, and gently draw the shoulder blades down the back (see fig. 7.45). Stay for five breaths, then repeat on the other side. Return to Dandasana. Be careful not to pull too hard on the strap. Tune in to the front edge of the bent knee, and be sure that it feels safe and comfortable. If there is any undue pressure on the front of the bent knee, either use two blocks or explore another option for this asana.

Figure 7.45

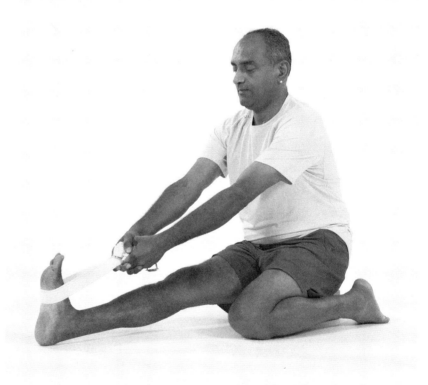

Janu Sirsasana A (Head-to-Knee Pose A)

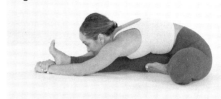

Figure 7.46

CHAIR VARIATION

Start off seated in a chair, and slide the hips to the front of the seat. Stack one or two blocks in front of the chair. Externally rotate the right hip joint, point the right knee out toward the side, and place the right foot on the blocks. Extend the left leg straight out, engage the quadriceps and muscles of the legs, and flex the left foot to ground through the left heel. Keep a little space between the blocks and the left leg. Align the torso and chest toward the left leg, place both hands on the left thigh, gaze forward, and pivot the hip joints to increase the hip flexion (see fig. 7.47). Maintain a relatively straight back and avoid overly rounding when folding forward. Stay for five breaths, then repeat on the other side. Return to seated.

FLOOR VARIATION

Start off seated on two folded blankets to elevate the hips. Externally rotate the right hip joint, point the right knee out to the side, and draw the right foot in as close to the pubic bone as possible. Place a block under the right knee to support the knee and relax the hip. Align the center of the chest forward toward the left knee, wrap a strap around the left foot, and hold the strap with both hands. Inhale and engage the muscles of the pelvic floor; draw the muscles of the lower abdomen in to support the spine and prepare for the pose. Exhale and fold into the hip joints to pivot slightly forward (see fig. 7.48). Allow a gentle rounding of the back muscles to elongate and stretch the muscles of the lower back. Gaze toward the left toes. Avoid overly rounding the back, pulling with the arms, forcing the right knee down, or otherwise exerting too much effort. Find a way to work the body with a deep sense of inner connection and compassion. Stay for five breaths, then repeat on the other side. Return to Dandasana.

Figure 7.47

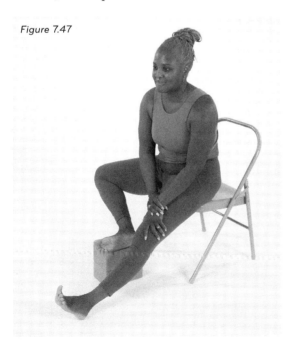

Figure 7.48

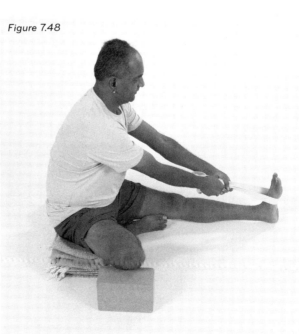

Figure 7.49

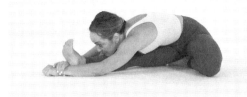

Janu Sirsasana B (Head-to-Knee Pose B)

CHAIR VARIATION

For the Chair Variation of this asana, repeat the option given for Janu Sirsasana A.

FLOOR VARIATION

Start off seated on a block to elevate the hips. Externally rotate the right hip joint, point the right knee out to the side, and draw the right foot in as close to the block as possible. Roll the right knee forward, and point the right foot. Elevate the hips to replicate the feeling of sitting on the foot that is indicated in the directions for Janu Sirsasana A. Align the center of the chest forward toward the left knee, wrap a strap around the left foot, and hold the strap with both hands. Inhale and engage the muscles of the pelvic floor; draw the muscles of the lower abdomen in to support the spine and prepare for the pose. Exhale and fold into the hip joints to pivot slightly forward (figs. 7.50 and 7.51). Allow a gently rounding of the back muscles to elongate and stretch the muscles of the lower back. Gaze toward the left toes. Place careful attention on the activation of the pelvic floor. The hamstring is elevated, allowing a deeper stretch but also placing it under a slightly increased stress. Avoid overly rounding the back, pulling with the arms, forcing the right knee down, or otherwise exerting too much effort. Find a way to work the body with a deep sense of inner connection and compassion. Stay for five breaths, then repeat on the other side. Return to Dandasana.

Figure 7.50

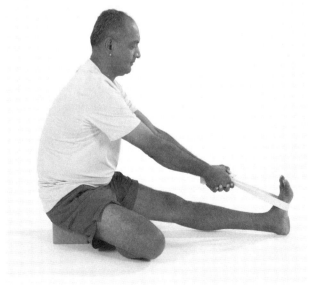

Figure 7.51

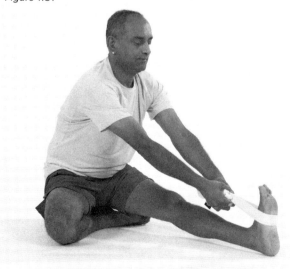

Janu Sirsasana C (Head-to-Knee Pose C)

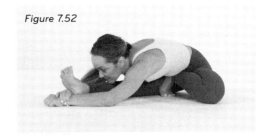

Figure 7.52

CHAIR VARIATION

Start off seated in a chair, and slide the hips to the front of the seat. Stack one or two blocks in front of the chair. Externally rotate the right hip joint, point the right knee out to the side, place the right foot on top and toward the inner edge of the blocks. Curl the toes back and ground down into the ball of the foot. Bend the right ankle, gently allow the knee to drop out to the side, and orient the right heel toward the left inner thigh. Extend the left leg straight out, engage the quadriceps and muscles of the legs, and flex the left foot to ground through the left heel. Keep a little space between the blocks and the left leg. Align the torso and chest toward the left leg, place both hands on the left thigh, gaze forward, and pivot the hip joints to increase the hip flexion (see fig. 7.53). Maintain a relatively straight back and avoid overly rounding while folding forward. Stay for five breaths, then repeat on the other size. Return to seated.

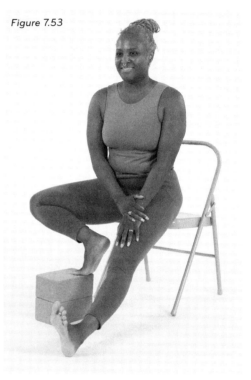

Figure 7.53

FLOOR VARIATION

Start off seated on a block to elevate the hips. Externally rotate the right hip joint, point the right knee out to the side, and draw the right foot in as close to the block as possible. Roll the right knee forward, and point the right foot. Elevate the hips to give the knee space. Curl the right toes back, and ground down into the ball of the foot. Bend the right ankle, gently allow the knee to drop out to the side, and orient the right heel toward the groin. Do not push the right knee down toward the ground. Align the center of the chest forward toward the left knee, wrap a strap around the left foot, and hold the strap with both hands. Inhale and engage the muscles of the pelvic floor; draw the muscles of the lower abdomen in to support the spine and prepare for the pose. Exhale and fold into the hip joints to pivot slightly forward

Figure 7.54

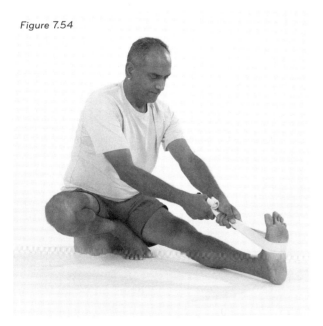

(see fig. 7.54). Allow a gentle rounding of the back muscles to elongate and stretch the muscles of the lower back. Gaze toward the left toes. Place careful attention on the activation of the pelvic floor. The hamstring is elevated, allowing a deeper stretch but also placing it under a slightly increased stress. Avoid overly rounding the back, pulling with the arms, forcing the knee down, or otherwise exerting too much effort. Find a way to work the body with a deep sense of inner connection and compassion. Stay for five breaths, then repeat on the other side. Return to Dandasana.

Try another option to focus more on grounding through the stretch in the toes. Start off in a kneeling position with both feet pointed and snuggled under the hips. Check this position to be sure that total knee closure feels comfortable. If it does not, then do not proceed. From a kneeling position, curl the toes under and sit on the feet. Extend the left leg forward, straighten the leg, and place weight in the left heel. Externally rotate the right hip joint, point the right knee out to the side, and keep sitting on the right heel. Place the hands on either side of the left leg and orient the torso forward toward the left knee (see fig. 7.55). The knee should be totally safe and protected while the stretching sensations remain localized in the toes and ankle. Gaze toward the right knee or the left toes. Stay for five breaths, then switch sides. Return to Dandasana.

Figure 7.55

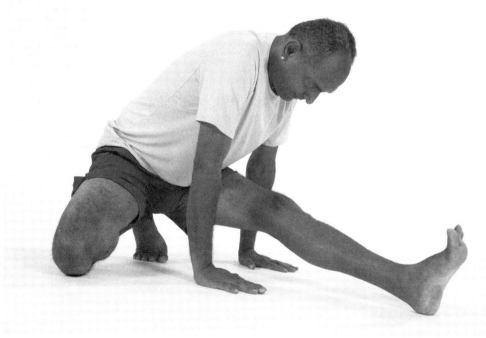

Marichasana A
(Pose Dedicated to Sage Marichi A)

CHAIR VARIATION

Start off seated in a chair, and stack two blocks in front of it. Align the legs hip-width apart. Place the right foot flat on top of the blocks and close the right hip joint. Slide to the front of the chair. Extend the left leg out, flex the foot, and engage the quadriceps. Hold on to the right knee with the right hand, and place the left hand on the left lower thigh. Inhale to prepare, engaging the pelvic floor and drawing the muscles of the lower abdomen in toward the spine. Exhale and fold the chest closer to the right leg, deepening the hip flexion (see fig. 7.58). Gaze forward. Stay for five breaths, then repeat on the other side. Return to seated.

Figure 7.56

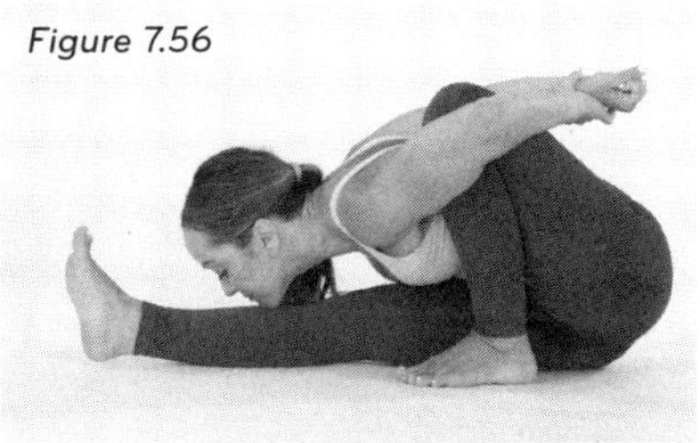

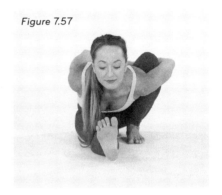

Figure 7.57

Figure 7.58

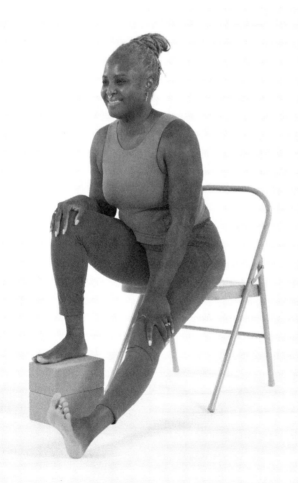

Figure 7.59

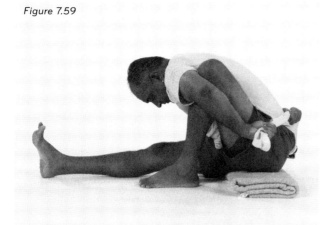

Figure 7.60

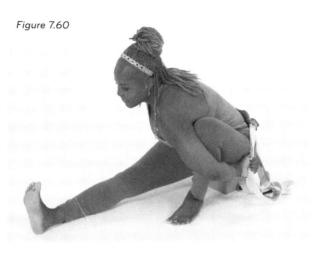

FLOOR VARIATION

Sit on a thickly folded blanket to lift the hips slightly and keep the pelvis grounded. Elevating the hips encourages a gentle hip flexion and increases the pivot forward inside the pelvis that assists with forward folding. Align the legs hip-width apart. Bend the right knee, keeping it in line with the right hip joint and maximizing the right hip joint's flexion. Slide the torso forward around the inside edge of the right thigh, and align the center of the chest toward the left knee. Internally rotate the right shoulder, and bend the right elbow down around the right shinbone. Hold a strap with the left hand and internally rotate the left shoulder to reach around the back toward the right hand. Allow both hands to grip the strap firmly. Inhale to prepare and create space along the core of the body. Exhale and allow the spine to fold forward, slightly entering a spinal flexion to facilitate deeper movement in the hips and lower back (see fig. 7.59). Allow the right ankle to bend as weight gently pours into the right foot. Gaze either down toward the left leg or forward toward the left toes. Stay for five breaths, then repeat on the other side. Return to Dandasana.

This asana can also be done seated on a block or a higher pelvic support (see fig. 7.60). Adjust the height according to what works for the body while paying careful attention to the alignment pointers. It is also possible to use the same hand position as shown in the Chair Variation from seated to avoid binding the arms. This could be advisable if the shoulders are sore or injured.

Marichasana B
(Pose Dedicated to Sage Marichi B)

CHAIR VARIATION

Start off seated on a chair. Repeat the Chair Variation from either Ardha Baddha Padmottanasana Chair Variation or Marichasana A. Focus on the combination of external rotation of one hip joint while deepening the hip flexion of both hip joints. Explore how much forward fold feels comfortable (see fig. 7.63). Be creative and explore the foundational elements of the asana. Maybe there's another alternative that works better than these suggestions.

Figure 7.61

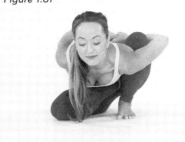

Figure 7.62

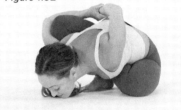

Figure 7.63

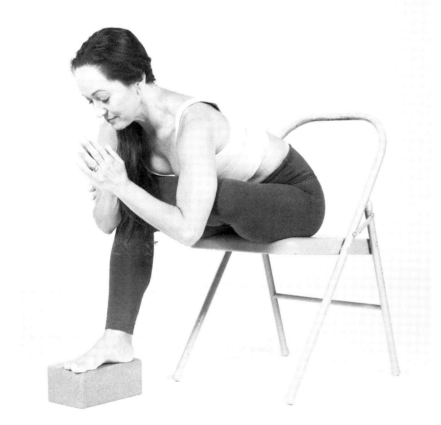

Figure 7.64

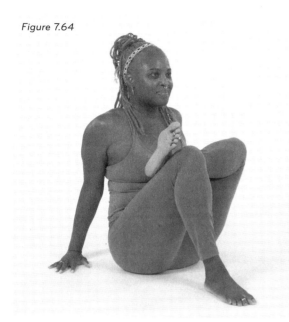

Figure 7.65

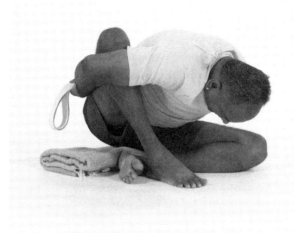

FLOOR VARIATIONS

Start off seated in Dandasana. Externally rotate the left hip joint and make a number 4 shape with the legs by stacking the left foot on the lower outer edge of the right thigh. Bend the right knee in toward the chest and allow the pelvis to rotate gently into a very slight posterior tilt. Place the hands slightly behind the pelvis. Inhale to create space, engage the muscles of the pelvic floor, and lift the rib cage away from the pelvis. Exhale to gently shift the torso closer to the thigh and deepen the hip flexion (see fig. 7.64). Gaze forward at a single point. Stay for five breaths, then repeat on the other side. Return to Dandasana.

Sit on a thickly folded blanket to lift the hips slightly and keep the pelvis grounded. Elevating the hips encourages a gentle hip flexion and increases the pivot forward inside the pelvis that assists with forward folding. Externally rotate the left hip joint and fold the left foot under the right thigh. Bend the right knee and align the right foot just in front of the left ankle. Slide the torso forward around the inside edge of the right thigh and align the center of the chest between both knees. Internally rotate the right shoulder, and bend the right elbow down around the right shinbone. Hold a strap with the left hand, and internally rotate the left shoulder to reach around the back toward the right hand. Allow both hands to grip the strap firmly. Inhale to prepare and create space along the core of the body. Exhale and allow the spine to fold forward, slightly entering a spinal flexion to facilitate deeper movement in the hips and lower back (figs. 7.65 and 7.66). Allow the right ankle to bend as weight gently pours into the right foot while keeping a sense of grounding through the back of the right hip. Gaze down. Stay for five breaths, then repeat on the other side. Return to Dandasana.

Figure 7.66

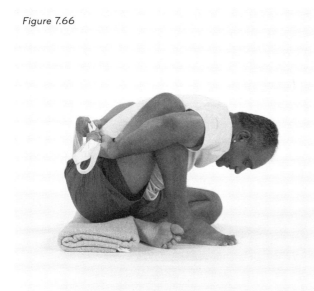

Figure 7.67

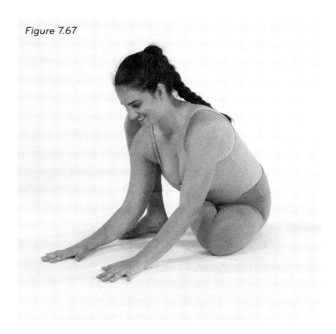

For an option with Padmasana without the bind, try this. Start off seated in Dandasana; fold the left leg into a half-lotus position using an external rotation of the left hip joint. Situate the left foot along the right hip crease and activate the left foot in a demi-pointe position; allow the left knee to point about forty-five degrees out to the side. Bend the right knee up toward the torso, and align the right foot with the outer edge of the right hip joint. Shift the pelvis and body weight forward until the left knee rests comfortably on the floor, but do not force the left knee down. If the knee fails to comfortably rest on the floor or if there is pain in the knee, then try one of the other options already listed. Pivot even farther forward until the torso slides around the inner edge of the right thigh. Place both hands on the floor. Inhale to prepare, lengthen the spine, engage the pelvic floor, and draw the muscles of the lower abdomen in toward the spine. Exhale and settle the weight into the hands (see fig. 7.67). Gaze down and slightly forward. Stay for five breaths, then repeat on the other side. Return to Dandasana.

Figure 7.68

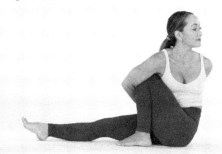

Figure 7.69

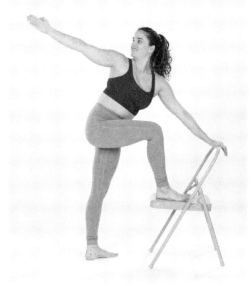

Marichasana C
(Pose Dedicated to Sage Marichi C)

CHAIR VARIATION

Start off in a chair. Stand up and turn toward the chair. Align the feet hip-width apart. Inhale and place the right foot on the seat of the chair. Lift the ribs away from the hips, engage the pelvic floor, and draw the muscles of the lower abdomen in toward the spine. Stabilize the muscles of the left leg, and reach the hands down toward the backrest of the chair. Inhale again and open the torso toward the right, extending the left arm around toward the back (see fig. 7.69). Maintain as much space as possible between the ribs and the hips and between the vertebrae. This variation can be used for any twist, including Utthita Parsvakonasana B from the standing poses in chapter 6.

Try the next option from seated on the chair. Stack two blocks in front of the chair. Align the legs hip-width apart. Place the right foot flat on the blocks, and close the right hip joint a little. Rest the hips in the middle of the seat. Extend the left leg out, ground into the left foot, engage the quadriceps, and firmly root down with the left leg. Gently hold on to the backrest with the right hand. Reach the left arm around the outer edge of the right thigh. Inhale to prepare, lift the ribs away from the hips, engage the pelvic floor, and draw the muscles of the lower abdomen in toward the spine. Exhale and twist around the spinal axis with a gentle rotation along the center line of the body (see fig. 7.70). Concentrate the twist primarily in the thoracic spine. Allow a slight internal rotation of the right hip joint and maintain stability in the pelvis to avoid twisting or rotating in the sacrum or lower back. If there is a bit of side bending or lateral stretching and the chest folds a bit toward the right, that is okay as long as it feels good. Avoid dumping weight into the lower back, and lengthen out through the top of the head. Resist the temptation to pull on the chair and force the body into a twist. Use the backrest as a resting point for the arms, and let the core of the body do the work of the asana. Gaze toward the right. Stay for five breaths, then repeat on the other side. Return to seated.

Figure 7.70

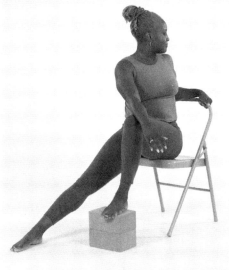

FLOOR VARIATION

Sit on a thickly folded blanket to lift the hips slightly and keep the pelvis grounded. Elevating the hips encourages a gentle hip flexion and increases the pivot forward inside the pelvis that assists with forward folding. Bend the right knee and guide the right foot toward the front edge of the blanket. Extend the left leg, engage the quadriceps, root down through the left heel, and draw the left femur slightly back into its socket. Settle the right hand on the floor slightly behind the pelvis, and hug the right leg by nestling the right shinbone in the crease of the left elbow. Inhale to create space, lengthen the spine, engage the pelvic floor, draw the muscles of the lower abdomen in, and float the rib cage away from the hips. Exhale to

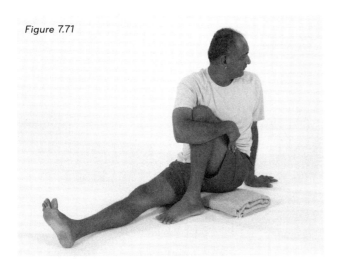

Figure 7.71

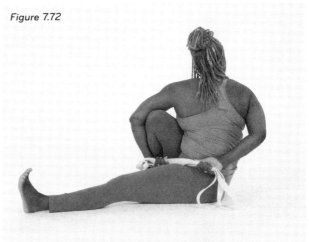

Figure 7.72

twist gently around the spinal axis, fold the torso gently toward the right thigh, and deepen the right hip flexion (see fig. 7.71). Look gently toward the right.

If the center of the chest moves comfortably around the right thigh and the body weight naturally shifts forward, it might be helpful to remove the blanket and use a strap to bind the hands. After taking a few breaths to settle into the inner work of the asana, place a strap on the left hip crease. Inhale again and slide the left hand around the right thigh by internally rotating the left shoulder, laterally moving the torso around the thigh and twisting the spinal axis. Hold the strap gently. Exhale and reach the right hand around the back, internally rotate the right shoulder, and clasp the other end of the strap (see fig. 7.72).

There is a temptation to hike the hips, but the asana is best practiced with the hips settled on the floor. The pelvis forms the foundation of the asana, while the torso performs the lifting and bending components. Twisting the hips too much may cause discomfort in the sacrum, lower back, or hip joints. While internally rotating the right hip joint assists with twisting, be careful not to overdo it. Avoid dumping weight into the lower back, and keep the body weight shifting forward. It may feel hard to breathe here, but that is merely the twist applying pressure on the organs of the abdomen and doing the inner work of purification. Remain calm and sensitive to the body's limits. Choose which option works best. Stay for five breaths, then repeat on the other side. Return to Dandasana.

Figure 7.73

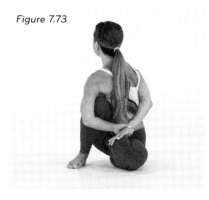

Figure 7.74

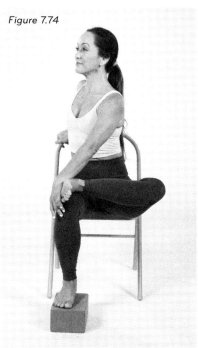

Figure 7.75

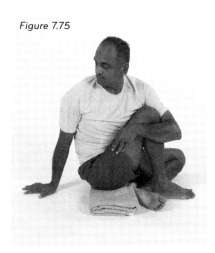

Marichasana D
(Pose Dedicated to Sage Marichi D)

CHAIR VARIATION

Start off seated on a chair. Repeat the Chair Variation for Ardha Baddha Padmottanasana to prepare. Gently hold on to the backrest with the right hand. Reach the left arm toward the right knee. Inhale to prepare, lift the ribs away from the hips, engage the pelvic floor, and draw the muscles of the lower abdomen in toward the spine. Exhale and twist around the spinal axis with a gentle rotation along the center line of the body (see fig. 7.74). Concentrate the twist primarily in the thoracic spine. Allow a slight internal rotation of the right hip joint and maintain stability in the pelvis to avoid twisting or rotating the sacrum or lower back. If there is a bit of side bending or lateral stretching and the chest folds a little toward the right, that is okay as long as it feels good. Avoid dumping weight into the lower back, and lengthen out through the top of the head. Resist the temptation to pull on the chair and force the body into a twist. Use the backrest as a resting point for the arms, and let the core of the body do the work of the asana. Gaze toward the right. Stay for five breaths, then repeat on the other side. Return to seated.

FLOOR VARIATION

Sit on a thickly folded blanket or a block to lift the hips slightly and keep the pelvis grounded. Elevating the hips encourages a gentle hip flexion and increases the pivot forward inside the pelvis that assists with forward folding. Externally rotate the left hip joint and fold the left foot under the right thigh. Bend the right knee, and align the right foot just in front of the left ankle. Settle the right hand on the floor slightly behind the pelvis, and hug the right leg by nestling the right shinbone in the crease of the left elbow. Inhale to create space, lengthen the spine, engage the pelvic floor, draw the muscles of the lower abdomen in toward the spine, and float the rib cage away from the hips. Keep both sitting bones grounded on the blanket. Exhale to twist gently around the spinal axis, fold the torso gently toward the right thigh, and deepen the right hip flexion (see fig. 7.75). Look gently toward the right. Stay for five breaths, then repeat on the other side. Return to Dandasana.

Figure 7.76 *Figure 7.77* *Figure 7.78*

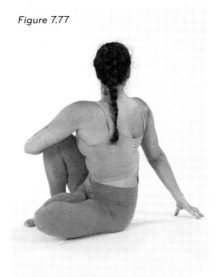
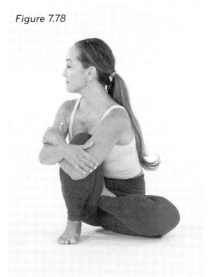

OTHER OPTIONS

If the center of the chest moves comfortably around the right thigh and the body weight naturally shifts forward, it might be helpful to use a strap to bind the hands. After taking a few breaths to settle into the inner work of the asana, place a strap on the left hip crease. Inhale again and slide the left arm around the right thigh by internally rotating the left shoulder, laterally moving the torso around the thigh and twisting the spinal axis. Hold the strap gently with the left hand. Exhale and reach the right arm around the back, internally rotate the right shoulder, and clasp the other end of the strap with the right hand (see fig. 7.76).

For an option with Padmasana but without the bind, try this. Start off seated in Dandasana, and fold the left leg into a half-lotus position using an external rotation of the left hip joint. Situate the left foot along the right hip crease; activate the left foot in a demi-pointe position, and allow the left knee to point about forty-five degrees out to the side. Bend the right knee up toward the torso, and align the right foot with the outer edge of the right hip joint. Shift the pelvis and body weight forward until the left knee rests comfortably on the floor, but do not force it down. Allow the sitting bones to lift off the ground. If the left knee fails to rest comfortably on the floor or if there is pain in the knee, then try one of the other options already listed. Inhale to prepare, lengthen the spine, engage the muscles of the pelvis floor, and draw the muscles of the lower abdomen in toward the spine. Keep the right arm extended back behind the body to help shift body weight forward (see fig. 7.77). Stay here for a few breaths and check in with the body. If the body feels good, then shift the weight forward fully into the strength of the pelvic floor, and hug the right thigh with both arms fully wrapping around the right shin (see fig. 7.78). Gaze to the right. Stay for five breaths, then repeat on the other side. Return to Dandasana

Figure 7.79

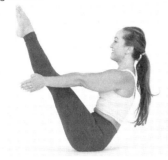

Figure 7.80

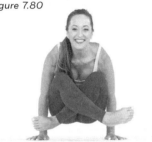

Navasana (Boat Pose) and Tolasana (Scales Pose)

CHAIR VARIATION

Start off seated on a chair. Slide the hips toward the back of the chair, and allow the back to be lightly supported by the backrest. Engage the muscles of the pelvic floor, draw the muscles of the lower abdomen in toward the spine, and keep a sense of elongation through the chest. Inhale and bend the knees as the legs lift off the ground. Place the hands under the knees to support the hip flexion (see fig. 7.81). Gaze forward. Shift as much weight off the backrest and into the core of the body as feels comfortable (see fig. 7.82). Stay for five breaths, then hold Purvottanasana (see fig. 7.37) for one breath to release the front of the hips.

It might also be fun to practice the lifting movement between two chairs. Align two chairs slightly wider than shoulder-width apart. Place a block on the floor between them, slightly forward from the front feet of each chair. Place the hands on the outer front edge of the chair seats and step up onto the blocks. Keep the arms straight, fold the front body into a deep

Figure 7.81

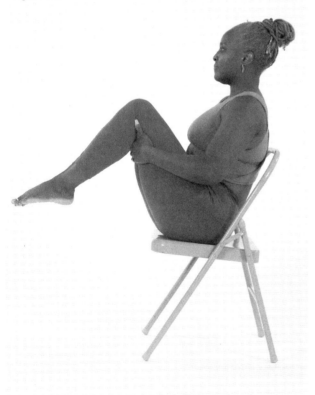

Figure 7.82

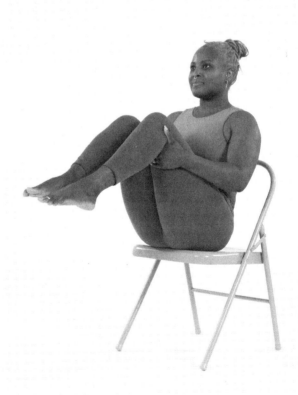

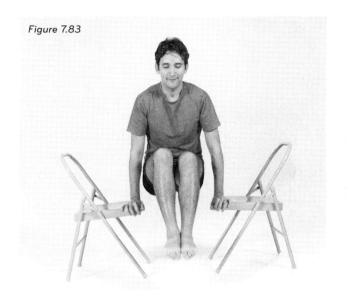

Figure 7.83

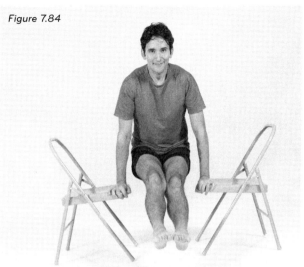

Figure 7.84

spinal flexion, activate the muscles of the shoulder girdle, firm the chest, and draw the knees to lift off the blocks or pour weight into the hands (see fig. 7.83). Slowly straighten the legs as the body feels stronger and more stable (see fig. 7.84). Stay for one breath, then continue with repetitions of Navasana. Repeat both Navasana and the Tolasana a total five times. Return to seated.

FLOOR VARIATION

Start off seated on a folded blanket. Settle the sitting bones slightly under the hips, and allow the pelvis to have a very gentle posterior tilt. Align the feet hip-width apart and bend the knees approximately ninety degrees. Avoid leaning too far back or dumping weight into the lower back. Engage the muscles of the pelvic floor, draw the muscles of the lower abdomen in toward the spine, and keep a sense of elongation through the chest. Inhale, bend the knees, and lift the arms to shoulder height (see fig. 7.85). If this feels unsafe, try holding the thighs just under the knees as shown in the Chair Variation for this asana. If the body feels stable, consider lifting the feet off the ground by engaging the muscles of the pelvic floor and increasing the hip flexion (see fig. 7.86). Keep the knees either hip-width apart or gently pressed together. As a way to practice straightening the legs, try holding the ankles or lower calf muscles with both hands while the knees are bent. Deepen the forward fold by drawing the femurs into their sockets, lengthening the chest, and then straighten the legs. Be careful not to push out with the legs or the abdomen. Engage the quadriceps, and roll the shoulder blades down the back. Choose which seated option best supports the work of the practice. Stay for five breaths. Then inhale to lift up for one breath.

Figure 7.85

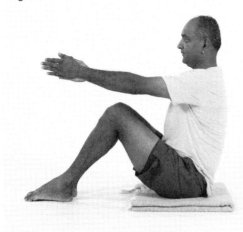

Figure 7.86

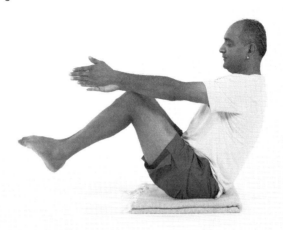

For Tolasana, place two blocks on the floor slightly in front of the hips shoulder-width apart. Cross the shinbones and lift the knees up into the chest. Explore which block height works best to facilitate the lifting movement. Engage the muscles of the shoulder girdle, fire up a firm front-body activation, and place the hands on the center of the blocks. Root down through the hands; send the shoulders forward and slightly down to lift the hips back and slightly up (see fig. 7.87). Let the goal be to lift only the hips at first. Do not worry about the feet remaining on the floor. Remember to hold this lift for one full inhalation, then return to seated and continue from there. While some other styles of yoga may practice Tolasana with the legs folded in Padmasana, in Ashtanga Yoga the lift-ups during Navasana should only be attempted with crossed legs. Repeat both Navasana and the lift a total of five times. Return to seated.

Figure 7.87

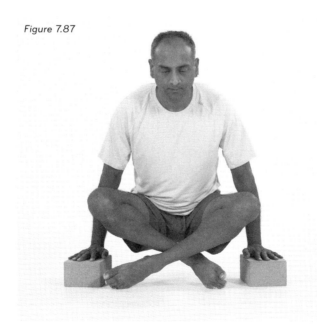

Bhujapidasana (Shoulder Pressing Pose)

CHAIR VARIATION

Start off seated on a chair. Scoot the hips to the front of the seat. Externally rotate the hips about forty-five degrees, and point the knees about ninety degrees away from each other. Place both hands on the lower thighs and lean slightly forward so weight begins to transfer into the legs. Inhale to prepare, activate the muscles of the pelvic floor, and draw the muscles of the lower abdomen in toward the spine. Exhale and place both hands in prayer position and bend forward (see fig 7.90). Explore the limits of hip flexion and forward folding, but don't push to surpass the limit. Gaze toward the nose. Stay for five deep breaths, then return the hands to the thighs. Exhale and stay here to settle and stabilize. Return to seated.

Figure 7.88

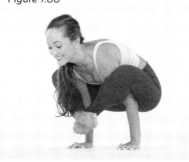

Figure 7.89

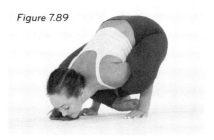

Figure 7.90

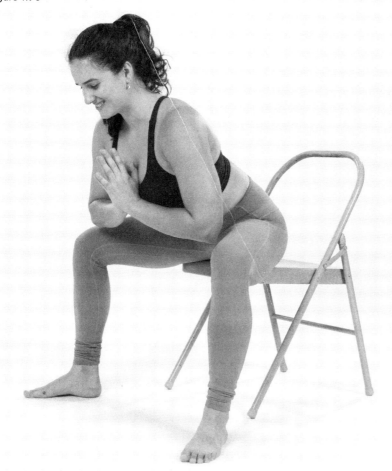

Figure 7.91

Figure 7.92

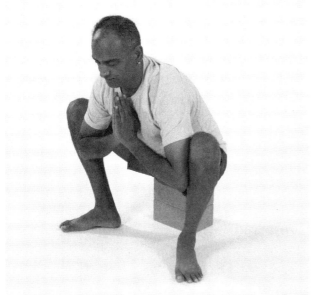

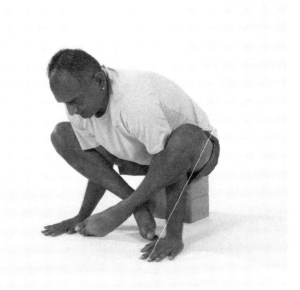

FLOOR VARIATION

Start off seated on two blocks with knees bent. Externally rotate the hips about forty-five degrees, and point the knees about ninety degrees away from each other. Place both hands in prayer position, snuggle the torso down between the thighs, and stabilize the shoulder girdle. Inhale to prepare, activate the muscles of the pelvic floor, and draw the muscles of the lower abdomen in toward the spine. Exhale and gently transfer the weight forward to increase hip flexion (see fig. 7.91). Gaze slightly down. Stay for five breaths. Either return to Dandasana or explore some of the options for Bakasana (Crow Pose) as part of the transition to complete the movement.

If external rotation and hip flexion are easily accessible, try another option. Still sitting on the blocks, place the hands on the floor shoulder-width apart, bend the elbows, fold the legs around the upper arms, and cross the ankles. Exhale to dip the chest slightly forward and pitch a little weight into the shoulders (see fig. 7.92). Be careful not to overdo it, and avoid trying to push too much weight forward or off the blocks. This option is a wonderful way to practice this asana when the wrists are injured.

Kurmasana (Tortoise Pose)

CHAIR VARIATION

Start off seated on a chair. Scoot the hips to the middle of the seat. Allow the legs to be just slightly wider than hip-width apart so there is just enough space for the torso to slide between the thighs. Avoid turning the hips too far out. Instead, actively draw the inner thighs toward each other. Place two blocks on the floor shoulder-width apart and slightly in front of the chair. Inhale to create space, engage the muscles of the pelvic floor, and draw the muscles of the lower abdomen in toward the spine. Exhale to fold forward, reach toward the blocks with the hands, relax the muscles of the back, draw the lower ribs in gently, and gaze down between the blocks or forward beyond the blocks (figs. 7.94 and 7.95). If it feels uncomfortable to place the hands on the blocks, then consider placing the hands on the thighs as in the previous pose. Explore the limits of hip flexion and forward folding, but don't push to surpass the limit. Stay for five deep breaths, then return to the hands to the thighs. Exhale there to settle and stabilize. Either return to seated or proceed immediately to Supta Kurmasana.

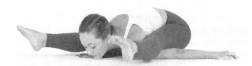

Figure 7.93

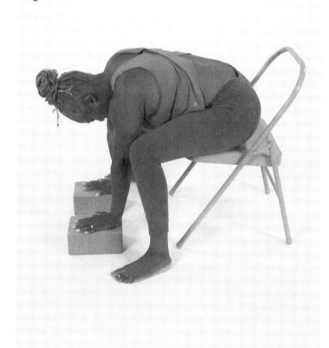

Figure 7.94

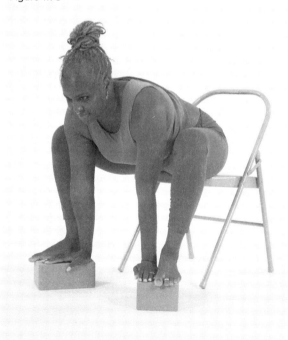

Figure 7.95

Figure 7.96

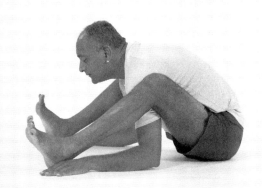

Figure 7.97

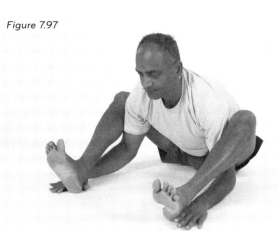

FLOOR VARIATION

Start off in Dandasana. Spread the feet slightly wider than hip-width apart, but be careful not to go too wide. Engage the legs, flex the feet, draw the muscles of the lower abdomen in toward the spine, and activate the pelvic floor. Inhale to create space and prepare. Exhale as the torso slides between the thighs; the knees stay bent while the elbows reach toward the ground. Slide the hands beside the heels, firm the chest, press the shoulders back against the legs, snuggle the thighs around the shoulders and upper torso, and stabilize the collarbones (figs. 7.96 and 7.97). Gaze toward the nose and keep the neck elongated and reaching forward. Stay for five breaths. Either return to Dandasana, proceed immediately to Supta Kurmasana, or explore one of the options for Bakasana as part of the transition to complete the movement. Keeping the knees bent is an accessible way to work the asana without placing too much pressure on the collarbones or the hamstrings. However, once the elbows firmly touch the ground, it is appropriate to start thinking about straightening the arms and legs.

Supta Kurmasana (Sleeping Tortoise Pose)

Figure 7.98

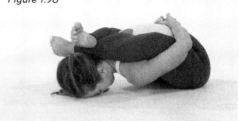

CHAIR VARIATION

Continue immediately from Kurmasana. Place a second chair, footrest, or some other supportive object in front of the chair. Slide toward the back of the seat. Lift both feet and place them on the second chair. Externally rotate both hip joints and allow the knees to drop out to the sides. Bring the heels and the bases of the little toes toward each other—touching them together or not—and gently turn the soles of the feet up. Inhale to create space, engage the muscles of the pelvic floor, and draw the muscles of the lower abdomen in toward the spine. Exhale to fold forward, reach toward the feet with the hands, relax the muscles of the back, draw the lower ribs in gently, and gaze toward the feet (see fig. 7.99). Stay for five breaths, then return to seated. Note that it may be more comfortable to try this asana on a sofa or bed. Explore what works best to support the practice.

FLOOR VARIATION

Continue immediately from Kurmasana. Place a chair directly in front of the body and stabilize the feet of the chair. Inhale to create space, engage the muscles of the pelvic floor, and draw the muscles of the lower abdomen in toward the spine. Place both feet on the front edge of the seat of the chair. Externally rotate the hip joints, bring the soles of the feet together, and point the knees out to the sides. Inhale to fold forward, reach toward the front legs of the chair with the hands, slide the torso between the thighs, relax the muscles of the neck and back, draw the lower ribs in gently, and gaze down at the floor (see fig. 7.100).

Figure 7.99

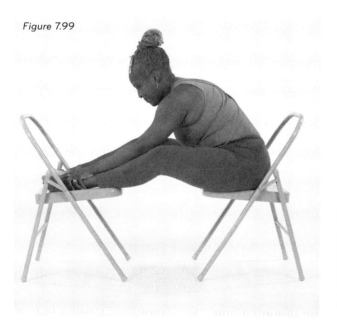

Figure 7.100

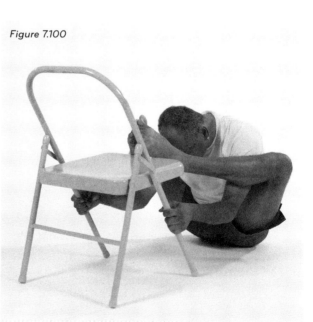

Figure 7.101

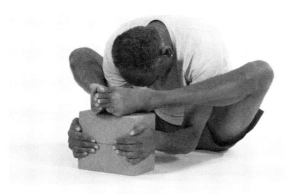

Figure 7.102

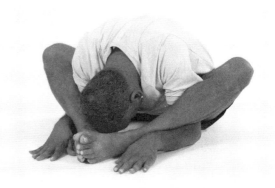

Figure 7.103

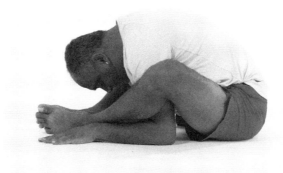

OTHER OPTIONS

Try this same principle with two blocks instead of a chair. Stack two blocks directly in front of the body. Place both heels on the blocks and follow the same alignment cues as those outlined for the Floor Variation. Instead of reaching toward the front legs of the chair with the hands, reach for the blocks under the feet and between the legs (see fig. 7.101).

Try the pose without the blocks or the chair. Place both feet together in a diamond shape. Slide the hands under the ankles and rest the hands around the feet. Follow the same alignment cues as those already outlined; rest the head down toward the insteps of the feet (see fig. 7.102). Avoid overly rounding the spine, pulling on the feet, or forcing the body in any manner. Gaze toward the nose. Note that the head may remain floating even as it reaches toward the soles of the feet (see fig. 7.103).

Once the head rests firmly on the floor under the feet and in front of the two blocks, try binding the hands around the back, first without a strap. Internally rotate the shoulders; reach the arms around the thighs and the hands up along the lower back toward the sacrum. As the arms find their position, clasp the hands (see fig. 7.104). Maintain a firm grip on the hands,

Figure 7.104

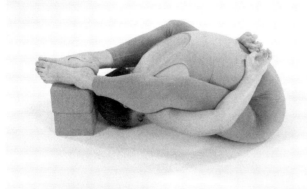

Figure 7.105

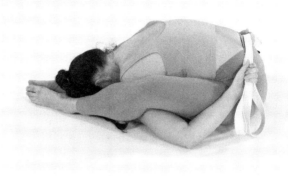

Figure 7.106

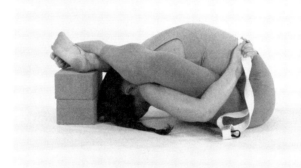

and actively push back into the weight of the legs to stabilize and protect the collarbones.

Now try it with a strap but without the blocks. If the head comfortably touches the ground behind the heels, it may be advisable to bind the hands with the assistance of a strap. Maintain the spinal flexion and the support of the bandhas. Keep the head as close to the ground as possible. Clasp a strap with one hand. Internally rotate the shoulders; reach the arms around the thighs and the hands up along the lower back toward the sacrum. As the arms find their position, clasp the strap with both hands and engage the shoulder girdle (see fig. 7.105). Maintain a firm grip on the strap and actively push back into the weight of the legs to stabilize and protect the collarbones. Use the strap in combination with any of the other options already outlined to best support the body during the practice. Try crossing the feet over each other on both blocks and holding a strap with the hands to support the chest and collarbones (see fig. 7.106).

Stay for five breaths. Either return to Dandasana or explore one of the options for Bakasana as part of the transition to complete the movement.

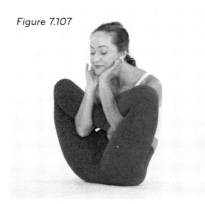

Figure 7.107

Garbha Pindasana (Womb Embryo Pose)

CHAIR VARIATION

Start off seated on a chair. Slide the hips toward the back of the seat. Lean gently on the backrest. Engage the pelvic floor and the muscles of the lower abdomen. Inhale to create space, lengthen the back muscles, draw the lower ribs in, lightly round the spine, cross the shinbones, and lift the legs off the floor and in toward the chest. Reach around the body and hold the tops of the feet with the hands (see fig. 7.108). Gaze forward. Balance here for five breaths. Gently rock back and forth in the chair. Inhale to lean slightly forward. Exhale to lean slightly back. Be careful not to fall off the chair or destabilize the chair itself. Proceed immediately to Kukkutasana (Rooster Pose).

FLOOR VARIATION

Start off seated on the floor. Engage the pelvic floor and the muscles of the lower abdomen. Inhale to create space, lengthen the back muscles, draw the lower ribs in, lightly round the spine, cross the shinbones, and lift the legs off the floor and in toward the chest. Reach around the body and hold the tops of the feet with the hands (see fig. 7.109). Gaze forward or toward the nose.

Figure 7.108

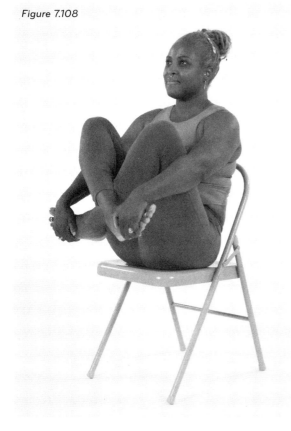

Figure 7.109

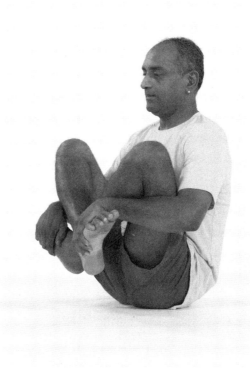

Figure 7.110

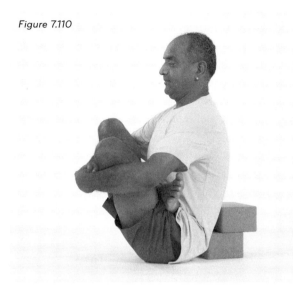

Figure 7.111

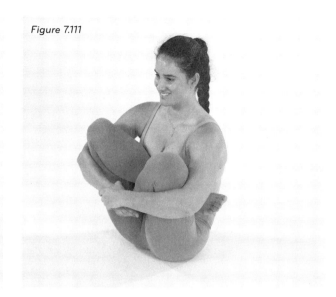

OTHER OPTIONS

Even if Padmasana is accessible, balance may still be a challenge. Stack two blocks a little behind the body. Inhale and fold the legs up into full lotus position using the external rotation of both hip joints. Gently tuck the tailbone, maintain activation of the bandhas, and fold the thighs in toward the body. Lean a little weight onto the blocks and reach the arms around the legs to clasp the hands if working with Padmasana. If clasping the hands is not accessible, then hold on to the thighs. If Padmasana is not accessible, then each hand should hold the opposite foot (see fig. 7.110). Gaze forward and balance for five breaths. If the balance feels stable, try this without the blocks (see fig. 7.111).

Figure 7.112

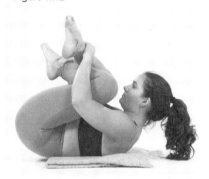

The next component of this asana is often referred to as "rounding," where the body rocks up and down using the strength of the pelvic floor. It is absolutely crucial to keep the body tightly knit together if the rocking motion is practiced. Sometimes the spine may feel undue pressure during this motion, in which case it is best to avoid it or practice on several thick blankets (see fig. 7.112). To proceed with rounding, tuck the head in toward the chest. Exhale and rock back; inhale and roll up. Try this a few times while moving in the same position. Eventually it may be advisable to turn in a circle while rounding up and down, executing a 360-degree turn with the body (see fig. 7.113). This movement is considered very advanced, so it is best to begin with gentle rocking that gets the body acquainted with the proprioception necessary to safely practice this movement.

Figure 7.113

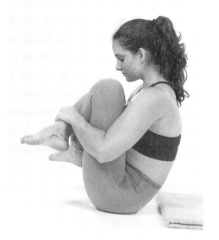

Figure 7.114

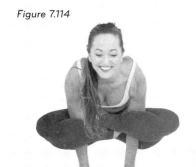

Kukkutasana (Rooster Pose)

CHAIR VARIATION

Proceed immediately from Garbha Pindasana. Either lift up into Purvottanasana or use the lift-up from Navasana between two chairs as outlined previously. Stay for five breaths and then return to seated.

FLOOR VARIATION

Proceed directly from Garbha Pindasana. Repeat the lifting position outlined in Navasana with two blocks. Stay for five breaths, then return to seated.

If Padmasana is accessible, then maintain the position and proceed with Kukkutasana, lifting up with the legs folded in full lotus. Place two blocks shoulder-width apart, slightly forward and on either side of the hips. Lift the legs into the chest and fold the thighs close to the body. Tuck the tailbone under and work into a spinal flexion. Draw the ribs down toward the hips, engage the front of the body, and prepare the shoulder girdle for weight bearing. Inhale to root down into the hands, pitch the shoulders slightly forward, and send the hips back (see fig. 7.115). Avoid hooking the feet on the arms or behind the forearms. Instead, focus on maintaining the knees at hip-height or higher by using the strength of the core, the legs, and the shoulders. The whole body is involved in this pose with a high level of activation. Stay for five breaths, then return to seated. If Padmasana is not accessible, then repeat the lift-up variation from Navasana that worked best.

Figure 7.115

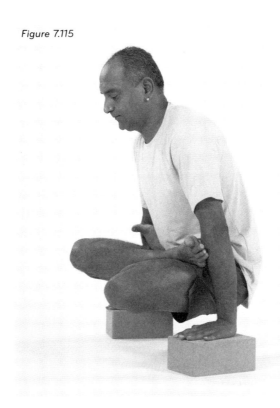

Baddha Konasana (Bound Angle Pose) A, B, and C

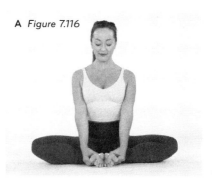

A *Figure 7.116*

CHAIR VARIATION

Start off seated on a chair, and stack two blocks slightly in front of it. Slide the hips toward the center of the seat. Externally rotate both hip joints, lift the feet onto the blocks, and allow the knees to fall out to the sides. Settle the hands on the knees or the lower portion of the tops of the thighs. Draw the muscles of the lower abdomen in, engage the muscles of the pelvic floor, and elongate the spine. Inhale to prepare. Exhale and gently tip the torso forward, pivoting at the hip joints (see fig. 7.119). Gaze toward the nose. Stay for five breaths. Exhale and round the back. Hold on to the knees, and tuck the chin in toward the spine. Stay for another five breaths. Inhale to return to the first position for one breath. Exhale again and return to seated.

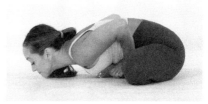

B *Figure 7.117*

Try a reclining variation using a chair, a wall, the back of a sofa, or the headboard of a bed. Start off in a reclining position. Externally rotate the hips, lift the feet onto the seat of the chair or any place on the object that feels supportive, and allow the knees to fall out to the sides. Use only the engagement necessary to keep the feet aligned with each other and maintain the external rotation of the hips (see fig. 7.120). Rest the hands by the hips. Close the eyes or gaze toward the nose. Stay for fifteen breaths or more, depending on the flow of the practice.

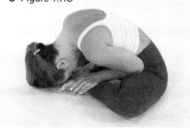

C *Figure 7.118*

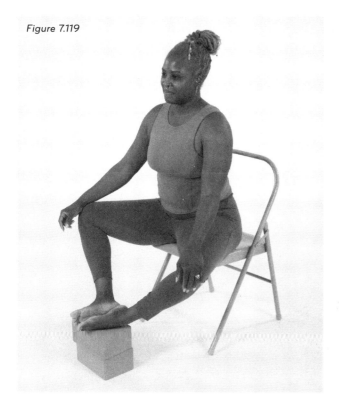

Figure 7.119

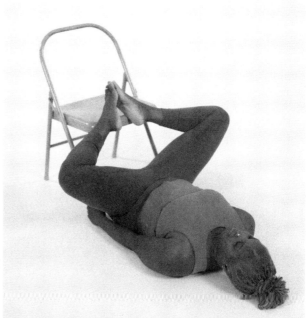

Figure 7.120

Figure 7.121

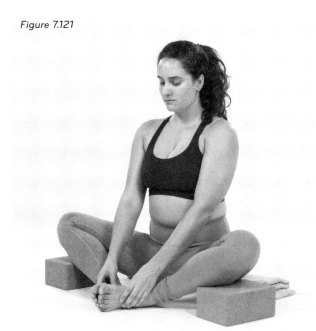

Figure 7.122

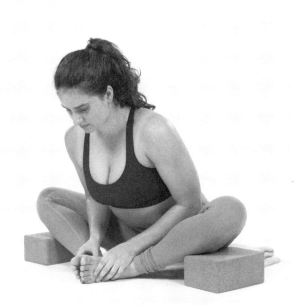

FLOOR VARIATION

Start off seated on a folded blanket. Externally rotate the hips and draw the feet in toward the pubic bone. Close the knee joints as tightly as possible, but do not force the knees to close or move toward the floor. Place a block under each knee to support it. Slide the fingers around the feet, holding the mount of the big toe with the thumb and the knuckles of the remaining toes with the fingers. Draw the muscles of the lower abdomen in, and engage the muscles of the pelvic floor. Inhale to lengthen the spine and create space between the ribs and the hips (see fig. 7.121). Exhale to pivot forward, folding at the hip joints (see fig. 7.122). Gaze toward the nose. Stay for five breaths, then proceed immediately to Baddha Konasana B. Round the back and rotate the tailbone under (see fig. 7.123). Gaze toward the nose, and maintain activation of the bandhas. Stay for five breaths. Inhale and return to the first position; settle for a moment before returning to seated.

Figure 7.123

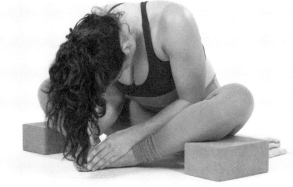

Upavistha Konasana
(Wide-Angle Seated Forward Bend) A and B

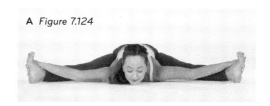

A *Figure 7.124*

CHAIR VARIATION

Start off seated in a chair. Place two blocks in front of the chair, wider than hip-width apart. Do not attempt the maximum distance between the blocks at the first attempt. Start with an accessible distance and work up from there over time. Place the feet on the blocks, root down through the heels, and flex the feet. Engage the muscles of the pelvic floor, draw the muscles of the lower abdomen in toward the spine, and create space for the forward fold. Inhale to prepare. Exhale and pivot forward, slide toward the front of the seat, fold forward, and reach the hands down along the legs toward the feet (see fig. 7.126). Stop at the beginning of a stretch through the legs and lower back. Do not pull on the legs or feet to try to force a deeper fold. Keep the legs as straight as possible, but also be willing to explore bending the knees if that helps facilitate deeper hip flexion.

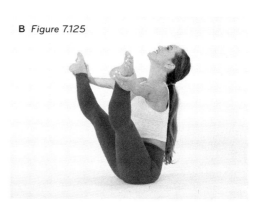

B *Figure 7.125*

Now try it with a strap. Place the feet on the floor, with the strap running under both insteps; open the thighs with a slight external rotation of the hip joints. Hold on to each end of the strap and bring the torso slightly forward over the thighs (see fig. 7.127). Gaze toward the nose or any point that encourages good balance. Be careful not to fall off the chair or slide too far forward. Stay for five breaths. Bend the knees, scoot the hips toward

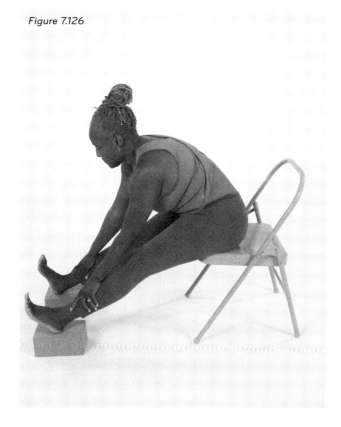

Figure 7.126

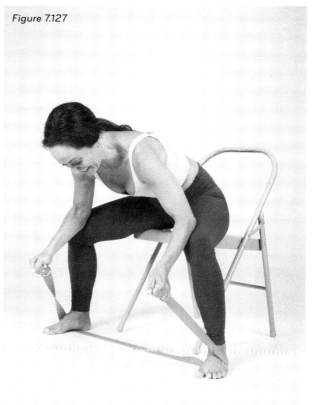

Figure 7.127

Figure 7.128

Figure 7.129

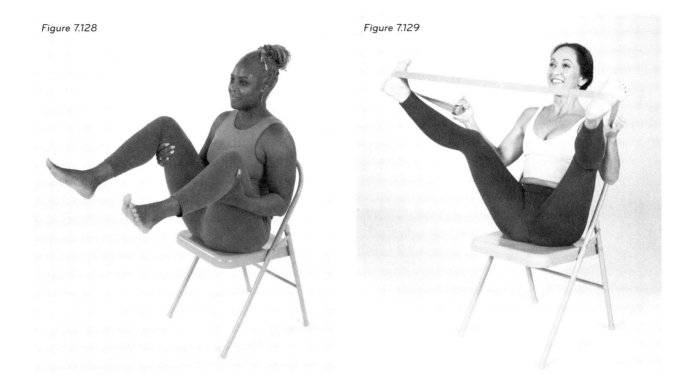

the back of the seat, hold the legs under the knees, and lift the thighs up toward the torso. Rest the upper back gently on the backrest of the chair, but avoid dumping weight into the lower back (see fig. 7.128). Try lifting up with the strap wrapped around the soles of the feet (see fig. 7.129). Be careful not to slide off the chair. If the seat of the chair is too small, try this transition on a sofa or a bed. Maintain strong activation in the core of the body. Gaze forward or slightly up. Stay for five breaths in balance, then return to seated.

FLOOR VARIATION

Start off seated in Dandasana. Open the legs out to the sides. Place a bolster in front of the body toward the pubic bone, and elevate the far end of the bolster with a block. Inhale and draw the muscles of the lower abdomen in toward the spine, engage the pelvic floor, and firm the quadriceps. Exhale and pivot forward, folding at the hip joints to bring the torso comfortably to rest on the bolster. Reach the hands down the legs and hold firmly on to either the ankles or the outsides of the feet near the little toes. Rest the chin on the bolster, and do not pull with the arms (see fig. 7.130). Try this without the bolster. Place the hands on the thighs, perhaps just above the knees. Do not pull or force the body down, but instead explore the natural limits of the forward fold. It is acceptance of where one is and the work of inner activation that support forward folding (see fig. 7.131). Now try it with a strap. Loop a strap around the arches of the feet and gently hold on to both ends of the strap with the hands. Bend the elbows slightly to stabilize the shoulder girdle (see fig. 7.132). Choose the variation that is best for the body. Gaze at the nose. Stay for five breaths.

Figure 7.130

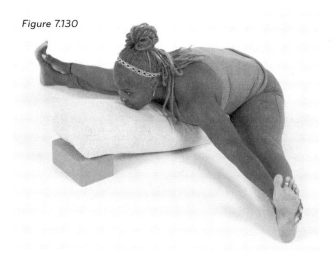

Figure 7.131

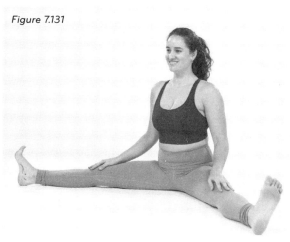

Figure 7.132

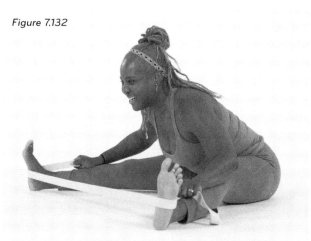

Figure 7.133

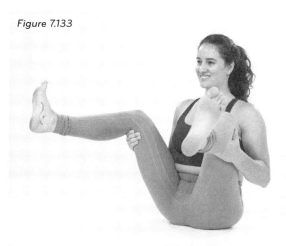

Proceed immediately to Upavistha Konasana B. Release the feet and inhale to lift the torso off the bolster. Bend the knees, rotate the tailbone under, and maintain the activation of the core and pelvic floor. Inhale to lift the legs off the ground, transfer a little extra weight down into the pelvis and come up to balance. Hold either underneath the knees, at the ankles, around the feet near the little toes, or any place on the leg that works for a firm grip with the hands (see fig. 7.133). If the strap option worked best for the first segment of this asana, then continue with the strap. Follow the same alignment cues in this instruction and balance with the strap wrapped around the feet (see fig. 7.134). Find the balance by aligning the torso with the center of gravity in the hips. Gaze upward. Stay for five breaths, then return to seated.

Figure 7.134

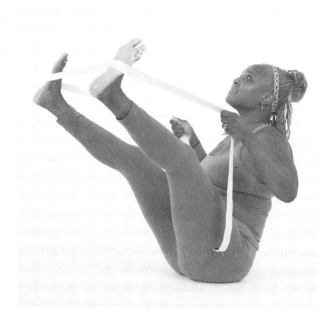

Figure 7.135

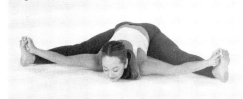

Figure 7.136

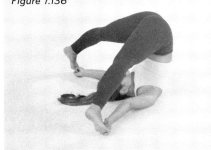

Supta Konasana (Reclining Angle Pose)

CHAIR VARIATION

Since this is a reclining pose, it may be advisable to skip any attempt at the prone variation of this asana and repeat the option outlined previously for Upavistha Konasana. In fact, unless the chair is very stable and wide enough to support the body, it may be more advisable to use a sofa or a bed for support for this pose. To adapt this asana, lie down on the seat of the chair, sofa, or bed. Inhale to draw the thighs up toward the body and extend the arms upward along the outsides of the legs to gently hold the calves. Gently curl the torso into a light spinal flexion and tuck the head in toward the chest. If the hands do not comfortably reach toward the lower legs, then use a strap. Stay for five breaths. Then lift up to the version of Upavistha Konasana that works best and stay for one breath (see figs. 7.137 and 7.138). Return to the same forward fold that worked for Upavistha Konasana A and settle for one breath before returning to seated.

Figure 7.137

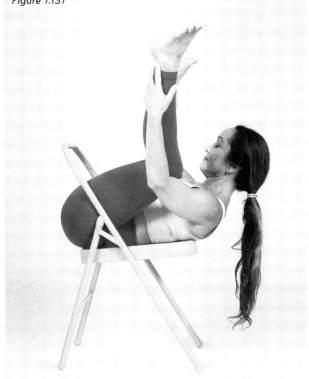

Figure 7.138

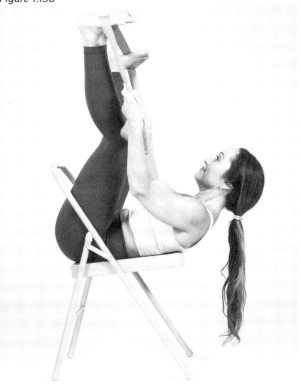

FLOOR VARIATION

Sometimes the full reclining movement of this asana can be too much for the neck. Instead of rolling all the way over, start off lying on the back without lifting the legs over the top of the head. With the back fully supported on the floor, inhale to lift the legs and fold the thighs in toward the chest as much as is comfortable for the body. Reach the hands up to support the legs, and place the hands behind the backs of the knees, along the shins, at the ankles, or holding the big toes or a strap around the feet (figs. 7.139 and 7.140). The legs can also be bent to give the hamstrings more space (see fig. 7.141). Stay for five breaths. Roll up to seated, either maintaining the hands' grip on the legs or releasing the legs in the process of coming up. Gently place the feet on the floor, extend the legs as much as is comfortable, and return to the same hand-to-leg grip established in the first portion of this asana (or a comfortable position practiced in Upavistha Konasana). Gaze toward the nose. Stay for one breath to settle, then return to seated.

Figure 7.139

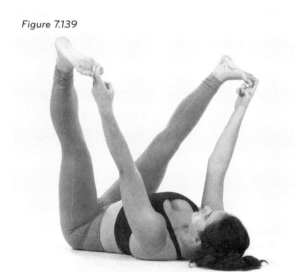

Figure 7.140

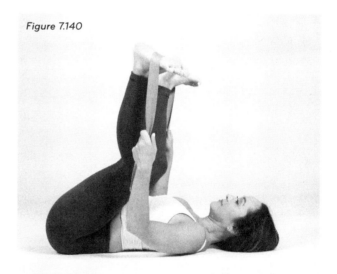

Figure 7.141

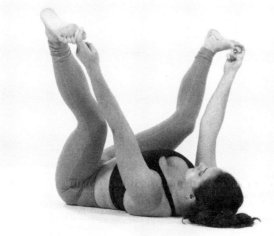

Figure 7.142

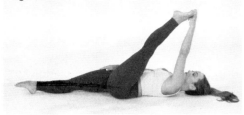

Figure 7.143

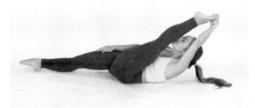

Figure 7.144

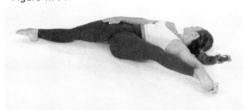

Supta Padangusthasana (Reclining Big Toe Pose)

CHAIR VARIATION

While seated on a chair, the practice of Supta Padangusthasana and Utthita Hasta Padangusthasana may appear very similar. However, the intention of these asanas diverges slightly in the traditional teaching. Utthita Hasta Padangusthasana is a balancing asana that works to strengthen the ability to balance under stress. Supta Padangusthasana improves flexibility and strength and is considered a more appropriate place to work on the principles of stretching and strengthening. So even if the same outward form of the asana is used, it is important to note the differences in approach and intention. While the figures here show the asana practiced with a straight leg, remember it is acceptable to bend the knee and focus exclusively on the hip flexion instead of emphasizing the stretch in the hamstrings and the backs of the legs. Always find the option that best supports personal practice.

Start off seated on a chair. Loop a strap around the arch of the right foot and hold on to the strap with the right hand. Inhale to lift the right leg; straighten the leg as much as is comfortable, settle the left hand on the natural waist, and stabilize the left leg. Lean lightly toward the back of the chair to replicate the supportive feeling of lying on the floor. Activate the muscles of the pelvic floor, draw the muscles of the lower abdomen in toward the spine, and lengthen the torso to create space. Gaze toward the right toes (see fig. 7.145). If this stretch is enough, then stay here for

Figure 7.145

Figure 7.146

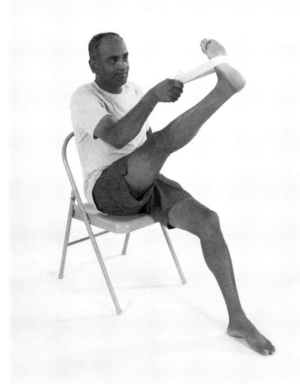

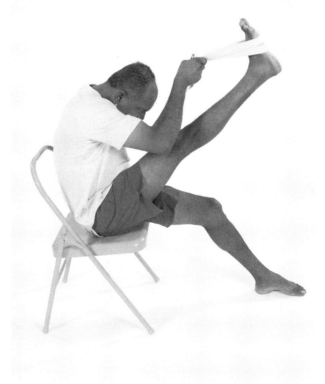

five breaths. If more of a stretch is possible, fold forward, drop the head slightly down toward the chin, lift the torso off the backrest, and align the center of the chest toward the right knee (see fig. 7.146). Exhale and settle into the pose for five breaths. Inhale and return to the initial position for one breath. Maintaining the activation of the pelvic floor, exhale and move the right leg out to the side, externally rotating the right hip joint, and gaze toward the left (see fig. 7.147). Stay for five breaths. Maintain firm activation of the core muscles, ground through the left leg, and stabilize the pelvis to avoid twisting the hips. After five deep breaths, inhale and return to the first position. Settle there or fold forward for one breath. Return to seated, then repeat on the left side. Return to seated again.

Figure 7.147

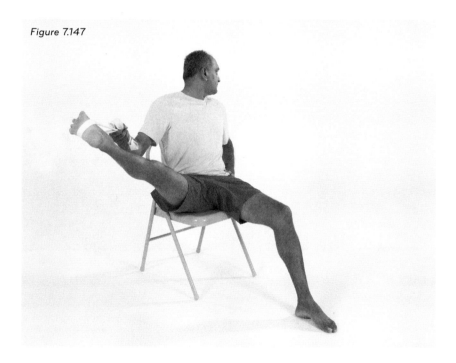

FLOOR VARIATION

Start off in Dandasana, then lie down. Bring both legs together and root down through the heels. Point the toes and place the hands on the tops of the thighs. Engage the pelvic floor, and draw the muscles of the lower abdomen in toward the spine. Inhale to lift the right leg. Explore the limits of hip flexion and forward fold flexibility. Based on the level of comfort and what feels best for the principles of the asana, either bend the knee and hold the shinbone (see fig. 7.148), bend the knee and hold the big toe, or wrap a strap around the middle of the foot to straighten the leg more (see fig. 7.149) Once the appropriate position is chosen, exhale to lift the torso toward the right leg. Align the center of the chest with the right knee, and gently tuck the chin in toward the chest to ease the burden on the back of the neck (see figs. 7.150 and 7.151). Gaze toward the nose or the right toes. Stay for five breaths. Inhale and return the torso and head to the ground.

Exhale and externally rotate the right hip joint to move the right leg gently out to the right. Continue whichever variation of the hip flexion and forward fold best supports the body's ability to do the inner work of the yoga practice. Keep the left hip and leg settled on the floor, and avoid hiking the hip or destabilizing the pelvis. Look toward the left. Keep the left hand in position on the left side of the body to help ground (see figs. 7.152 and 7.153). Stay for five breaths. Inhale and return the right leg to parallel alignment toward the center. Exhale and lift the torso again. Stay for one breath. Inhale and settle the torso and head back to the ground. Exhale and return the right leg to the floor. Repeat on the left side, then return to prone position. Either come up to seated or stay in the reclining position to continue the practice.

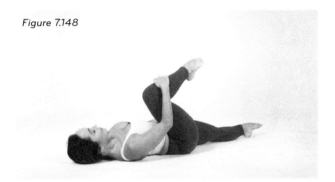

Figure 7.148

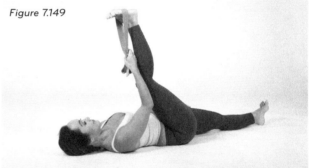

Figure 7.149

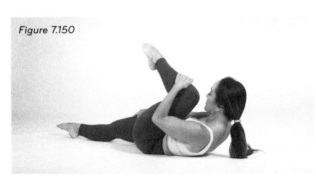

Figure 7.150

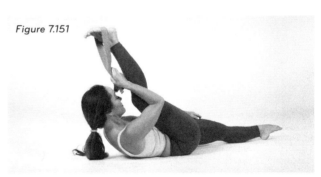

Figure 7.151

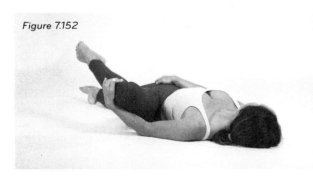

Figure 7.152

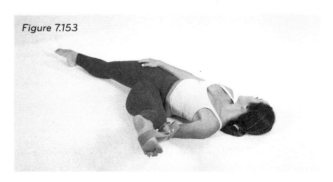

Figure 7.153

Ubhaya Padangusthasana
(Two-Foot Pose)

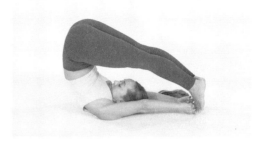

Figure 7.154

CHAIR VARIATION

Start off seated on a chair. Slide the hips toward the back of the seat and allow the back to be lightly supported by the backrest. Engage the muscles of the pelvic floor, draw the muscles of the lower abdomen in toward the spine, and keep a sense of elongation through the chest. Inhale and bend the knees as the legs lift off the ground. Hug the thighs in toward the body, wrapping the arms around the shinbones. Start off with the weight gently resting on the back of the chair. Stay for one breath. Inhale and shift the weight slightly forward, ground through the pelvis, and explore balancing on the chair. Gaze forward (see fig. 7.156). Stay for five breaths, then return to seated.

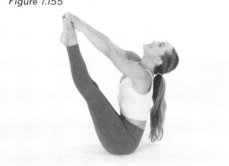

Figure 7.155

FLOOR VARIATION

Start off seated on the floor. Exhale to lie down. If the back is sensitive or sore, it may be useful to cushion the floor with a folded blanket or towel prior to reclining. Inhale and fold the legs up into the body. Explore whether it feels right to lift the legs over the head or whether it is better to remain lying on the back. If there are any preexisting neck injuries or weaknesses, it may be best to refrain from attempting to hoist the legs over

Figure 7.156

Figure 7.157

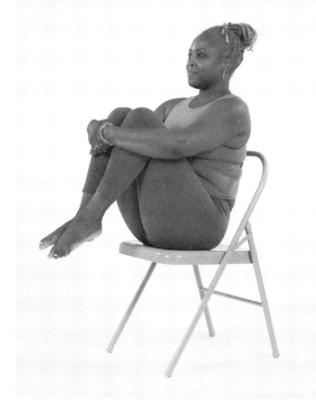

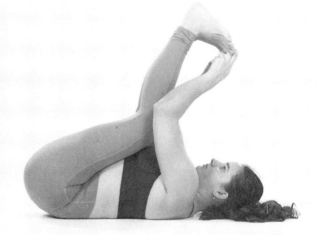

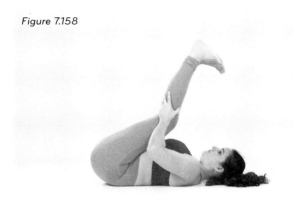

Figure 7.158

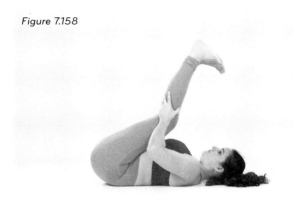

Figure 7.159

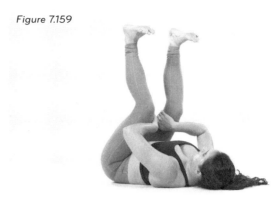

Figure 7.160

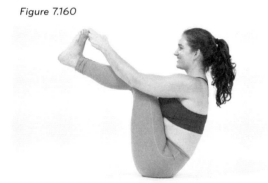

Figure 7.161

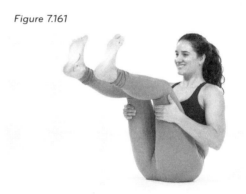

the head due to increased pressure on the neck. Engage the muscles of the pelvic floor, draw the muscles of the lower abdomen in toward the spine, lightly engage the shoulders, roll the spine slightly forward, and inhale in order to lift the legs and hips over the head. Whether reclining or with the legs over the head and settled on the floor, bend the knees and hold the big toes with the first three fingers of the hands (see fig. 7.157). Reaching toward the feet is accessible along both the inside and outside of the body (see figs. 7.158 and 7.159). For students with bigger bodies, hip injuries, or decreased forward-bend flexibility, it may feel more comfortable to reach for the toes along the inner edges of the thighs and use the thighs to gently draw the body closer together. For other students, it may feel more secure to reach for the toes along the outer edges of the thighs and use the strength of the arms to keep the legs tucked more closely together. Exhale here for one breath. Inhale and roll up to balance. Settle the body weight into the ground using the strength of the pelvic floor (see figs. 7.160 and 7.161). Do not attempt to balance on the sitting bones. Instead feel the space between the sitting bones and the tailbone, and allow the weight to inhabit this middle space. Avoid dumping weight into the lower back. Lift the ribs away from the hips, and gaze slightly up and forward. Draw the shoulder blades down the back, and avoid scrunching the neck. Stay for five breaths, then return to seated.

Urdhva Mukha Paschimottanasana (Upward-Facing Intense Stretch)

Figure 7.162

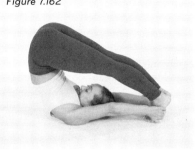

CHAIR VARIATION

Start off seated on a chair. Slide the hips toward the back of the seat and allow the back to be lightly supported by the backrest. Engage the muscles of the pelvic floor, draw the muscles of the lower abdomen in toward the spine, and keep a sense of elongation through the chest. Bend the knees to lift the legs off the ground and wrap a strap around the feet. Hold the strap with both hands, draw the shoulder blades down the back, and straighten the legs as much as is comfortable. Start off with the weight gently resting on the back of the chair. Stay for one breath. Then inhale and shift the weight slightly forward, ground through the pelvis, and explore balancing on the chair. Exhale and settle into the balance and forward fold. Gaze forward (see fig. 7.165). Stay for five breaths, then return to seated.

Figure 7.163

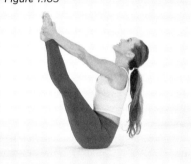

Figure 7.164

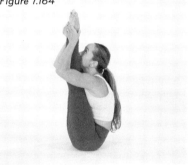

Figure 7.165

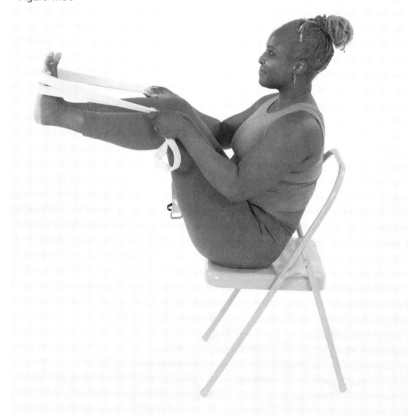

Figure 7.166

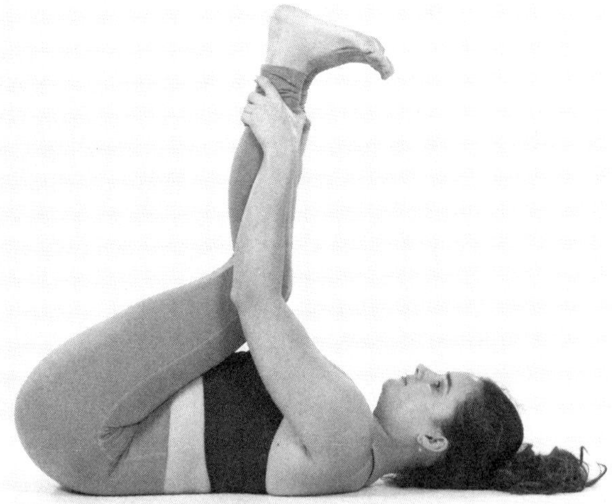

Figure 7.167

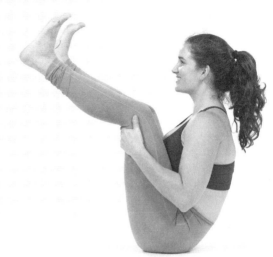

FLOOR VARIATION

It is absolutely acceptable to repeat the instructions listed for Ubhya Padangusthasana for this pose as well. However, it is also an option to make some small adjustments to work in a slightly different manner.

Start off seated on the floor. Exhale to lie down. If the back is sensitive or sore, it may be useful to cushion the floor with a folded blanket or towel prior to reclining. Inhale and fold the legs up into the body. Explore whether it feels right to lift the legs over the head or whether it is better to remain lying on the back. If there are any preexisting neck injuries or weaknesses, it may be best to refrain from attempting to hoist the legs over the head due to increased pressure on the neck. Whether from reclining or with the legs over the head and settled on the floor, bend the knees and either hold on to the ankles or wrap a strap around the feet (see fig. 7.166). Exhale here for one breath. Inhale and roll up to balance. Settle the body weight down into the ground using the strength of the pelvic floor (see fig. 7.167). Do not attempt to balance on the sitting bones. Instead feel the space between the sitting bones and the tailbone, and allow the weight to inhabit this middle space. Avoid dumping weight into the lower back. Lift the ribs away from the hips, and gaze slightly up and forward. Draw the shoulder blades down the back, and avoid scrunching the neck. If the balance is established, then exhale and deepen the forward fold while maintaining the balance. Bend the elbows and draw the torso close to the thighs. Gaze slightly up and forward. Stay for five breaths, then return to seated.

Setu Bandhasana (Spinal Lift Bridge Pose)

Figure 7.168

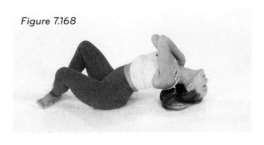

CHAIR VARIATION

Start off seated on a chair. Stack two blocks in front of the chair, slide the hips toward the front of the seat, and place both feet on the blocks. Externally rotate the hip joints, bend the knees, and draw the heels close together. Engage the legs, lift the pelvic floor, and draw the muscles of the lower abdomen in toward the spine. Inhale to lift the ribs away from the hips, settle the hands on the seat of the chair, extend the spine, and support the upper back and chest. Once the head and neck feel safe, gently look up (see fig. 7.170). Stay for five breaths, then return to seated.

Figure 7.169

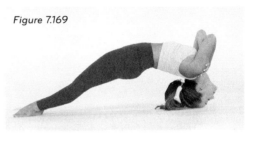

FLOOR VARIATION

The prepare position is often one of the best adaptations for this asana. Start off seated on the floor, then exhale to lie down. Inhale to lift the body into the prepare pose (see fig. 7.169 above); stay here for the entire asana. Externally rotate the hips, bend the knees slightly, and draw the heels in toward each other. Engage the legs, lift the pelvic floor, and draw the muscles of the lower abdomen in toward the spine. Inhale to lift the ribs away from the hips, extend the spine, and arch the neck to support the upper back and chest. Once the head and neck feel safe, lift the hands off the ground and cross the arms to hold each shoulder with the opposite hand.

Figure 7.170

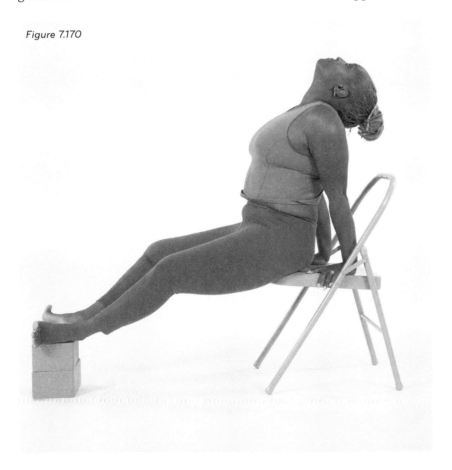

Figure 7.171

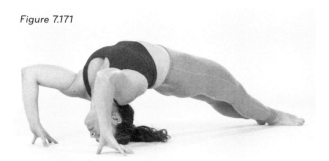

Figure 7.172

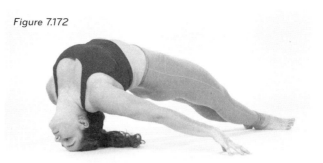

Gaze toward the nose. Do not rush to lift up; instead, stabilize the foundational elements of the asana to work on strength and flexibility. Stay here for five breaths, then return to reclining.

When there is a natural feeling of lift and stability in the body, place the arms either outstretched by the sides of the body or on either side of the head for support. Avoid pressing down with the arms; instead, use them to track the center line of the body. The strength to lift into this asana must originate from the muscles of the torso, neck, and legs. If the body feels safe, inhale to straighten and activate the leg and back muscles. Explore which hand position best supports the pose (see figs. 7.171 and 7.172). Stay for five breaths, gazing toward the nose. Exhale and bend the knees to return to the prepare position and then all the way back to reclining.

Try Setu Bandhasana with the support of a yoga wheel. Sit in front of the yoga wheel. Bend both knees, externally rotate the hip joints, and draw the heels in toward each other. Support the head, neck, and shoulders by resting the entire torso on the wheel. Maintain activation of the pelvic floor, and draw the muscles of the lower abdomen in toward the spine. Inhale and activate and straighten the legs to roll the body back over the wheel. Stop when the head touches the floor (see fig. 7.173). Use the arms as necessary for support throughout the movement. Feel the body entirely supported by the wheel yet activated to support the range of motion and keep the asana dynamic. Gaze toward the nose. Stay for five breaths, then return to seated by bending the knees and rolling out of the asana in the reverse of the manner used to enter it.

Figure 7.173

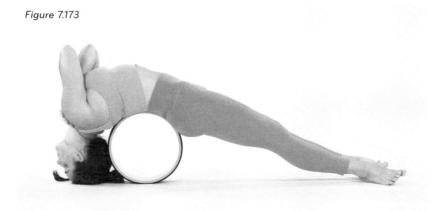

8

Intermediate Series / Second Series

THE INTERMEDIATE SERIES of Ashtanga Yoga is called *nadi shodhana* in Sanskrit and refers to the deep backbending, hip-opening, and strength-buidling asanas that provide one of the greatest challenges to the nervous system in the physical yoga asana practice. Many students find these obstacles to be insurmountable. Yet, there are many accessible options that open the bridge to some of the deeper benefits of the Intermediate Series. Backbending, for example, is a deeply therapeutic asana movement that is emphasized during the beginning of the Second Series. There is no other series of asanas within Ashtanga Yoga that systematically works to increase spinal extension and strength like the Intermediate Series, and providing an accessible entry point for these asanas increases the likelihood that more students will benefit from the practice. While some may find these adaptations to be heretical and contrary to the dogma of the practice, I believe that presenting accessible options for committed students on the path is the true heart of the lineage. Use these adaptations responsibly and maintain respect for yourself, the lineage, and the practice.

Figure 8.1

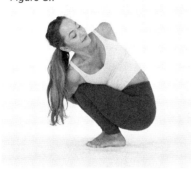

Pasasana (Noose Pose)

CHAIR VARIATION

Start off seated on a chair. Slide the hips forward toward the center of the seat. Open the knees to slightly wider than hip-width apart and firmly plant the feet on the floor. Place a block between the feet. Inhale and activate the muscles of the pelvic floor, draw the muscles of the lower abdomen in toward the spine, and create length and space between the ribs and hips. Avoid flopping the legs out to the side; use the inner thigh muscles to help the legs follow the line of the hips. Exhale and fold lightly forward, pivot at the hip joints, twist the torso at the thoracic spine, and reach the right hand down to press on the block (see figs. 8.2 and 8.3). Externally rotate the left arm and gaze up toward the left fingertips. Stay for five breaths, then repeat on the other side. Return to seated. Avoid twisting the hips, and use the strength of the core muscles to send weight back into the pelvis and stabilize the foundation.

Figure 8.2

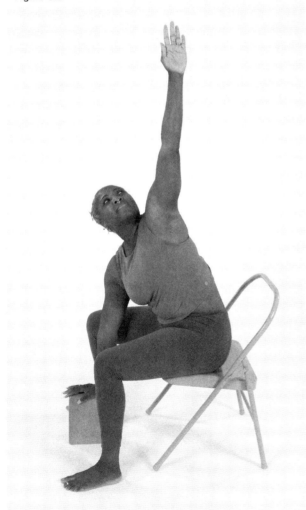

Figure 8.3

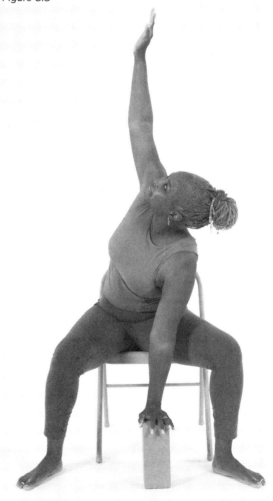

Figure 8.4

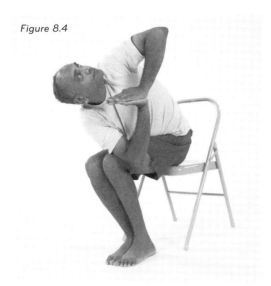

Figure 8.5

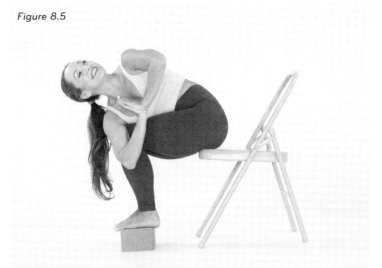

Figure 8.6

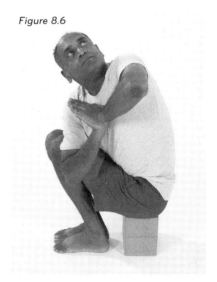

Try another option on the chair. Slide the hips toward the front of the seat. Keep both legs together, and activate the inner thigh muscles to draw the knees toward each other. Inhale and activate the muscles of the pelvic floor, draw the muscles of the lower abdomen in toward the spine, and create length and space between the ribs and hips. Exhale and fold deeply forward, pivot at the hip joints, and glide the torso around the outer edge of the left thigh. Twist the torso at the thoracic spine, drop the right shoulder down around the left knee, place the hands in prayer position at the center of the chest, and gaze over the left shoulder (see fig. 8.4). If the feet do not touch the ground easily, place a block under the feet for a solid foundation (see fig. 8.5). Avoid twisting the hips, allowing the knees to slide apart, or forcing the hip flexion. Stay for five breaths, then repeat on the other side. Return to seated.

FLOOR VARIATION

Figure 8.7

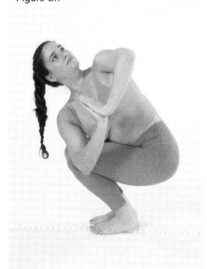

Start off seated in Dandasana. Stack two blocks behind the pelvis and sit comfortably on the blocks. Bend the knees and fold the legs to maximize hip flexion. Inhale and activate the muscles of the pelvic floor, draw the muscles of the lower abdomen in toward the spine, and create length and space between the ribs and hips. Exhale and fold deeply forward, pivot at the hip joints, and glide the torso around the outer edge of the left thigh. Twist the torso at the thoracic spine, drop the right shoulder down around the left knee, place the hands in prayer toward the center of the torso and gaze over the left shoulder (see fig. 8.6). Avoid twisting the hips, allowing the knees to slide apart, or forcing the hip flexion. Stay for five breaths, then repeat on the other side. Return to seated.

If Pasasana with the block feels comfortable, try it without the block. Activate the deep six hip rotator muscles, legs, pelvic floor, and core mus cles of the torso. Inhale to shift the weight onto the feet and maintain the balance and the twist (see fig. 8.7). If a comfortable squat is accessible, this

Figure 8.8   *Figure 8.9*

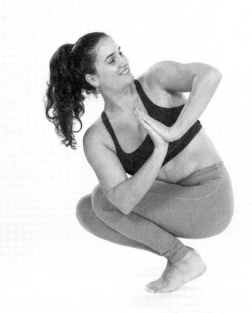

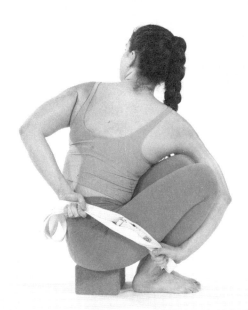

variation of the twist can be entered without the block by following the same alignment directions already given from a squat position.

If binding the hands feels approachable, then use a strap to access the movement safely. Seated on a block or in a steady squat with the hands in prayer position, release the hands and accentuate the lateral movement of the torso around the outer edge of the left thigh. Try balancing with the hands in prayer position (see fig. 8.8). Internally rotate the right shoulder, wrap the right elbow around the shinbones, and reach the right hand up toward the outer edge of the right thigh. Inhale and hold on to the strap with the left hand, elongate the collarbones, and gently loop the strap around the lower back and right hip crease so it falls toward the right hand. Gaze over the left shoulder. Once both hands have a firm grip on the strap, activate the shoulder girdle and settle into the pose for five breaths (see fig. 8.9). Repeat on the other side, then return to seated.

Krounchasana (Heron Pose)

CHAIR VARIATION

Start off seated on the chair. Slide the hips toward the front of the seat. Rest either the tips of the toes or the top of the foot on the floor, whichever feels more comfortable. If the right foot does not comfortably reach the ground, then use a block as a footrest. Thread a strap around the left foot and bend the left knee. Inhale and lift the left leg lightly off the ground, activate the muscles of the pelvic floor, draw the muscles of the lower abdomen in toward the spine, and engage the left quadriceps. Keep the shoulder blades drawn down the back, and exhale to fold lightly forward (see fig. 8.12). The left leg can remain bent or straight and can hover parallel to the ground or slightly higher, depending on what feels comfortable. Avoid dumping weight into the lower back to force the leg to lift. Stay for five breaths, then repeat on the other side. Return to seated. If this feels uncomfortable, return to the instructions given for Tiryang Mukha Ekapada Paschimottanasana.

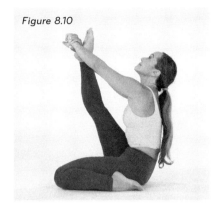

Figure 8.10

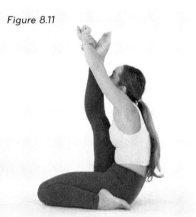

Figure 8.11

Figure 8.12

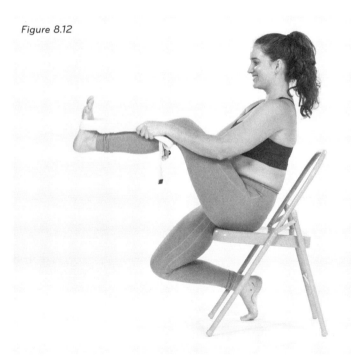

FLOOR VARIATION

Start off seated in Dandasana. Lift the hips onto a block so both sitting bones are firmly supported by the block. Internally rotate the right hip joint and fold the right leg back. Point the right toes near the outer edge of the block, and allow the knee to open slightly toward the right of the center line to give more space to the knee. Be sure that one block is sufficient to support the knee. If there is any pain around it, try sitting on two blocks or a larger object like a bolster, or practicing the preceding Chair Variation. Wrap a strap around the left foot and bend the left knee. Inhale to lift the

Figure 8.13

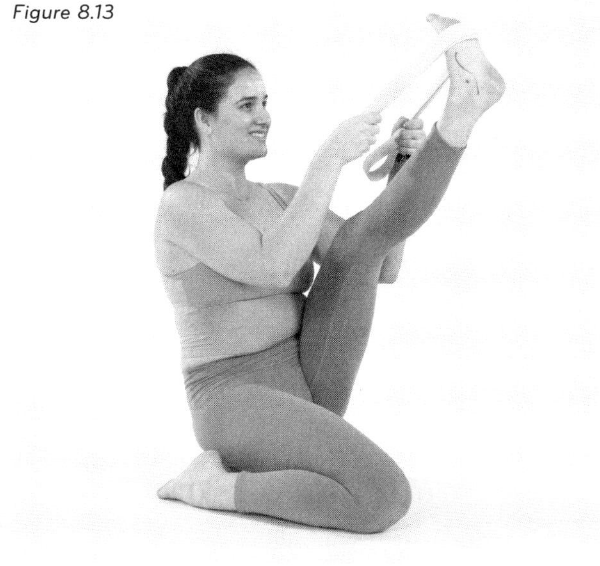

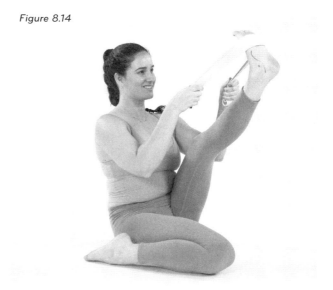

Figure 8.14

Figure 8.15

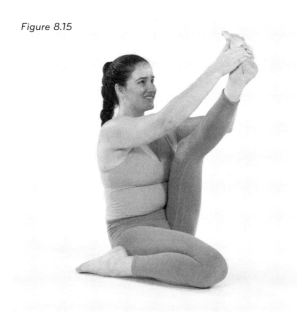

Figure 8.16

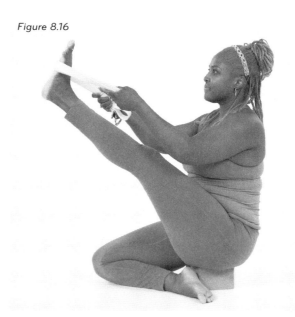

left leg off the ground, engage the muscles of the pelvic floor, and draw the muscles of the lower abdomen in toward the spine. Exhale to settle into the forward fold, draw the shoulder blades down the back, guide the body in toward the thigh, and straighten the leg as much as feels comfortable (see fig. 8.13). If the internal rotation of the right hip joint feels comfortable and there is no pressure on the knee, try this pose without the block (see fig. 8.14). Perhaps explore releasing the strap and working with a slightly bent knee to reach toward straightening the leg (see fig. 8.15), but be careful not to push too hard and damage the body. Remember there is no competition or comparison in yoga practice. Find what works for today and do not give up. In case the internal rotation of the hip joints is not accessible, try externally rotating the right hip joint to fold the leg in front of the block instead (see fig. 8.16). Gaze at the toes. Stay for five breaths, then repeat on the other side. Return to seated.

Shalabhasana A and B (Locust Pose A and B)

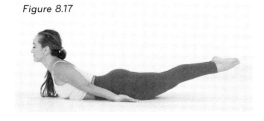

Figure 8.17

CHAIR VARIATION

Start off seated on a chair. Slide the body over to one side of the seat of the chair, lean down, and turn to come fully off the chair. Hold on to the seat and rest the forearms there. Allow a little weight to pour down into the forearms and engage the back muscles to lift the center of the chest. Gently place the torso on the seat of the chair, settling the weight in the space between the lower ribs and the hips. Hold on to the seat of the chair with both hands. Engage the pelvic floor, draw the muscles of the lower abdomen in toward the spine, firm the quadriceps, and activate the spinal muscles. Inhale and lift the legs, one by one, until they are hovering off the ground. If there is too much strain when both legs are off the ground (see fig. 8.19), alternate lifting one leg and then the other. Stay for a few breaths. Explore whether the body feels supported enough to change the hand position to either extending the arms back along the sides of the body or bending the elbows next to the chest (see fig. 8.20). While approaching Shalabhasana from a chair removes the need to get up from and down to the floor, do not assume that this pose is easy. The body is quite challenged in spinal extension. Remember to practice at a comfortable level of exertion.

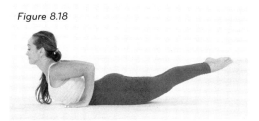

Figure 8.18

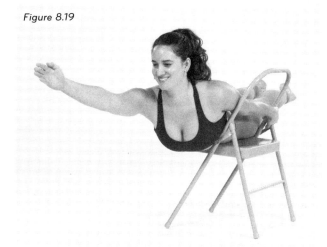

Figure 8.19

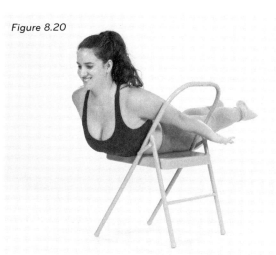

Figure 8.20

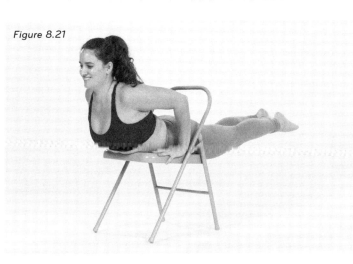

Figure 8.21

OTHER OPTIONS

Start off standing behind an open-back chair. Slide the torso onto the seat from the back and hold on to the seat of the chair with both hands. Bend the elbows and settle the lower ribs, abdomen, and pelvis on the seat. Engage the pelvic floor, draw the muscles of the lower abdomen in toward the spine, firm the quadriceps, and activate the spinal muscles. Inhale and lift the legs, one by one, until they are hovering off the ground (see fig. 8.21). If there is too much strain when both legs are off the ground, alternate lifting one leg and then the other.

FLOOR VARIATION

Start off in Adho Mukha Svanasana. Place a large, flat bolster or other supportive object in line with the body and a block or two between the feet. Inhale to come forward to Kumbhakasana and align the bolster with the chest. Engage the pelvic floor, draw the muscles of the lower abdomen in toward the spine, firm the quadriceps, and activate the spinal muscles. Exhale to lower onto the bolster. Place the feet on the blocks to lift the legs off the ground. Keep the head and chest elevated. Roll the shoulders forward, internally rotate the shoulder joints, turn the palms down, and reach the arms back along the sides of the body. Press all ten fingernail tips into the ground, lift the center of the chest and allow the neck to follow the line of the spine. Gaze toward the nose (see fig. 8.22). Stay for five breaths.

Maintaining the activation and alignment of all the muscles, gently change hand positions to proceed immediately to Shalabhasana B. Bend the elbows and form as close to a ninety-degree angle as possible with the arms. Turn the palms down to face the ground (see fig. 8.23). Pull—do not push—with the arms to create a sense of elongation through the spine and torso. Gaze at the nose. Stay for five breaths, then return to Adho Mukha Svanasana. Avoid craning the neck in an effort to feel more work. Instead, focus on elongating and strengthening. Explore potentially lifting the feet off the blocks, but avoid bending the knees or squeezing the back into any painful or compressive movements.

Figure 8.22

Figure 8.23

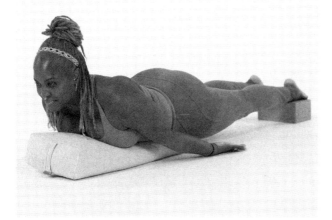

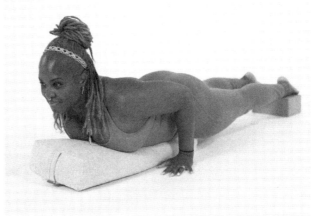

Bhekasana (Frog Pose)

Figure 8.24

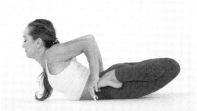

CHAIR VARIATION

Start off seated on a chair. Turn toward the left side of the seat and settle both feet firmly on the floor. Gently hold the backrest with the left hand, and slide the hips forward and slightly toward the right. Drop the right leg down toward the ground along the front of the chair to extend the right hip, and hold the right foot with the right hand. Engage the pelvic floor, and draw the muscles of the lower abdomen in toward the spine. Activate the back muscles to lift the ribs away from the hips. Internally rotate the right shoulder, and draw the right foot toward the outer edge of the right side of the hips to close the right knee joint and stretch the right quadriceps. Gaze either toward the nose or slightly up and forward at a single point (see fig. 8.25). Stay for five breaths, then switch sides. Return to seated. Be careful not to stress the knee or fall off the chair while working on this asana.

Figure 8.25

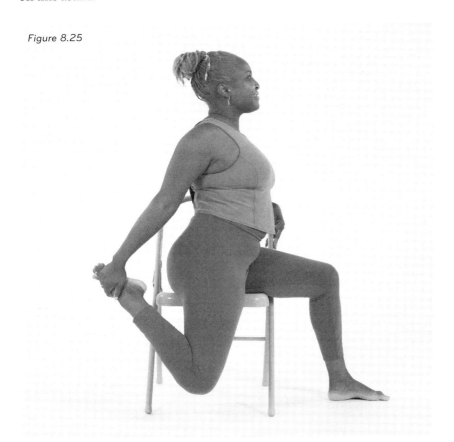

Figure 8.26

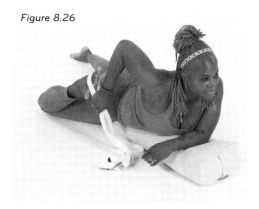

Figure 8.27

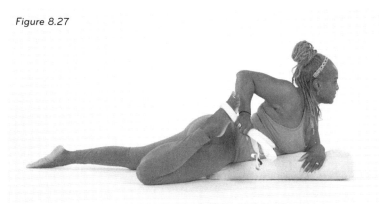

Figure 8.28

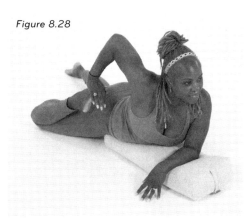

Figure 8.29

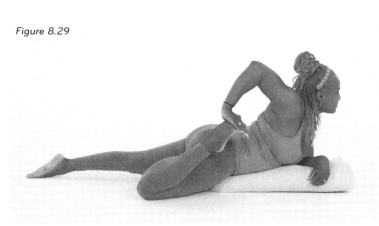

FLOOR VARIATION

Start off in Adho Mukha Svanasana. Place a large, flat bolster or other supportive object in line with the body. Inhale to come forward to Kumbhakasana, and align the bolster with the iliac crests at the front of the pelvis. Engage the pelvic floor, draw the muscles of the lower abdomen in toward the spine, firm the quadriceps, and activate the spinal muscles. Exhale to lower onto the bolster. Keep the left leg extended, and lift the upper portion of the torso to lift the upper back. Bend the left elbow in front of the body on the bolster, and rest the weight down into the left arm. Engage the upper back muscles to support the spine. Bend the right knee; reach back toward the right foot with the right hand, and wrap a strap around the right foot like a lasso. Engage the right arm to guide the right foot down around the outer edge of the right side of the hips; close the knee to elongate the quadriceps, the right hip, and the front of the pelvis (see figs. 8.26 and 8.27). If the right hand is close to the right foot, try the pose without the strap. Cradle the base of the right big toe between the right thumb and index finger. Close the right knee joint and flip the grip of the right hand so the fingers face forward and the heel of the hand rests on top of the knuckles of the right toes (see figs. 8.28 and 8.29). Avoid stressing the knee, and if any sharp pain appears, back off. Gaze either toward the nose or forward at a single point. Stay for five breaths, then switch sides. Hold the second side for five breaths, then inhale to lift up to Urdhva Mukha Svanasana and exhale back to Adho Mukha Svanasana.

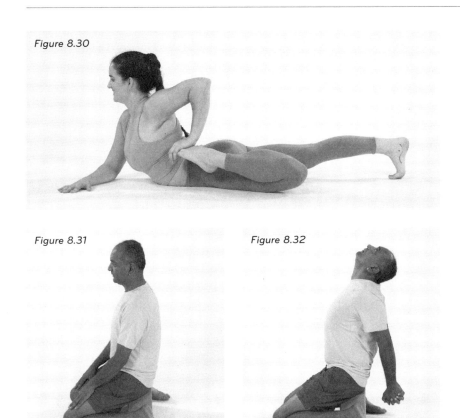

Figure 8.30

Figure 8.31

Figure 8.32

Explore Bhekasana without the bolster when the body feels ready. Apply the same directions with the body resting on the floor instead of the bolster (see fig. 8.30). Be very sensitive to the micromovements of the knee joint, and do not force the body in any way. Learn to listen to and respect the body's limits while remaining curious and open about the body's potential. Avoid craning the neck in an effort to feel more work.

OTHER OPTIONS

Explore an alternative if the knees are sore or painful. Seated on two blocks, practice Virasana (Hero Pose; see fig. 8.31). Internally rotate the hips and fold the legs back under the thighs. Align the feet on either side of the blocks. Let the hands rest on the thighs, lift the ribs away from the hips, engage the pelvic floor, and draw the muscles of the lower abdomen in toward the spine. Roll the shoulder blades down the back, and lift the center of the chest. Gaze toward the nose. To deepen the backbend, roll the shoulders forward, interlace the fingers behind the back, engage the back muscles, and gently tilt the head and neck upward. Gaze either toward the nose or up and forward at a single point (see fig. 8.32). Stay for five breaths, then return to seated.

Figure 8.33

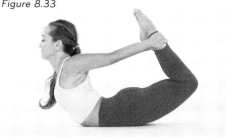

Dhanurasana (Bow Pose)

CHAIR VARIATION

To practice Dhanurasana from the chair, work with the earlier instructions for either Bhekasana or Shalabhasana. If getting up from and down to the floor is prohibited by a lack of knee flexion, then the following instructions for the Floor Variation may be practiced on a sofa or bed.

Figure 8.34

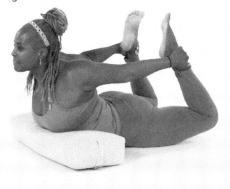

FLOOR VARIATION

Start off in Adho Mukha Svanasana. Place a bolster perpendicular to and toward the front of the mat. Exhale while lowering the body and placing the lower ribs on the bolster. Inhale and engage the pelvic floor, draw the muscles of the lower abdomen in toward the spine, lengthen the spine, and lift the chest. Bend the knees, and reach the hands back to clasp the ankles. Allow the legs to be slightly wider than, slightly less than, or about hip-width apart. Engage the quadriceps to lift the thighs slightly off the ground. Kick back with the strength of the legs and resist with the strength of the arms (see fig. 8.34). If reaching back toward the ankles is not accessible, use a strap looped around the ankles to assist. Internally rotate the shoulders and encourage the sternum to rise. Gaze at the nose. Stay for five breaths, then return to Adho Mukha Svanasana. Avoid craning the neck, and allow the neck and head to follow the arch of the back.

Figure 8.35

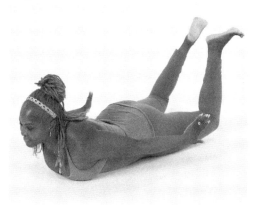

OTHER OPTIONS

Try the Floor Variation without the bolster. Start off in Adho Mukha Svanasana. Exhale as the stomach lowers to the floor. Inhale and engage the pelvic floor, draw the muscles of the lower abdomen in toward the spine, lengthen the spine, and lift the chest. Bend the knees and reach the hands back to clasp the thighs. Allow the legs to be slightly wider than, slightly less than, or about hip-width apart. Engage the quadriceps to lift the thighs slightly off the ground (see fig. 8.35). Stay here for a few breaths. Explore using a strap to bind the hands and ankles. Loop a strap around the ankles, and clasp each end with the hands (see fig. 8.36). Kick back with the strength of the legs and resist with the strength of the arms. Internally rotate the shoulders, and encourage the sternum to rise. Gaze toward the nose. Stay for five breaths, then return to Adho Mukha Svanasana. Avoid craning the neck, and allow the neck and head to follow the arch of the back.

Figure 8.36

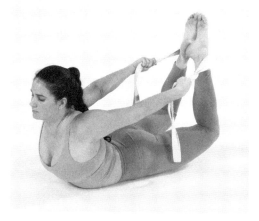

Parsva Dhanurasana (Side Bow Pose)

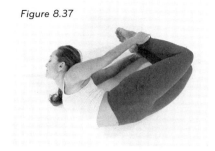

Figure 8.37

CHAIR VARIATION

Start off seated on the chair. Turn the body to the left side of the seat and scoot forward to the edge of the seat. Stabilize the left leg and move the body toward the front corner of the left side of the chair. Slide the right thigh off the chair and then lift it back and up onto the seat. Wrap a strap around the right ankle. Place the left hand on the left thigh. Inhale and engage the muscles of the pelvic floor, draw the muscles of the lower abdomen in toward the spine, lift the ribs away from the hips, and firm the shoulder girdle. Exhale and engage the back muscles to kick the right foot back (see fig. 8.38). Or try it without the strap (see fig. 8.39). Gaze forward at a single point. Stay for five breaths, then repeat on the other side.

Conclude the sequence of Parsva Dhanurasana by repeating the option that worked best for Dhanurasana. This Chair Variation is more challenging than it seems. Do not force the body, and always feel free to adapt the instructions to best support the practice. All students would benefit from practicing this variation as it opens the front of the hips and releases the psoas muscles to prepare for deeper backbending.

Figure 8.38

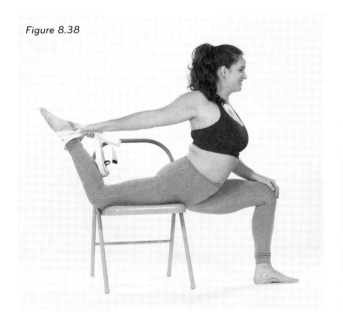

Figure 8.39

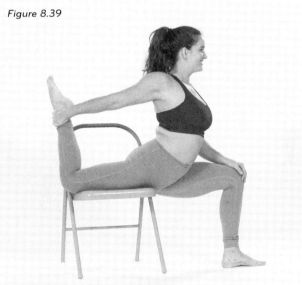

FLOOR VARIATION

To do the work of asymmetrical backbending in Parsva Dhanurasana, try using a variation of Dandayamana Bharmanasana (Balancing Table/Bird Dog Pose) as an alternative. Start on the hands and knees. Align the hands shoulder-width apart and the knees hip-width apart. Activate the pelvic floor, draw the muscles of the lower abdomen in toward the spine, and lift the ribs away from the hips. Work the opposite sides of the body. Inhale and extend the left arm and right leg. Externally rotate the left shoulder,

Figure 8.40

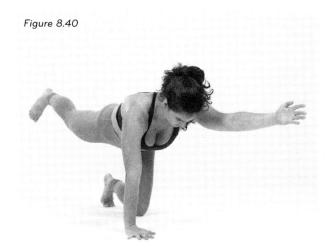

Figure 8.41

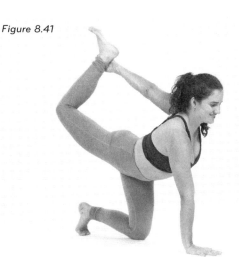

and engage the right quadriceps and open the front of the left hip (see fig. 8.40). Gaze down. Stay for five breaths. Bend the right knee and reach the left hand back to grasp the right ankle. Once the grip is firmly established, engage the right leg and the back muscles to create more space between the vertebrae (see fig. 8.41). Use a strap to make the binding more accessible (see fig. 8.42). Gaze at the nose. Stay for five breaths, then repeat on the other side. Conclude the sequence of Parsva Dhanurasana by repeating the option that worked best for Dhanurasana.

Figure 8.42

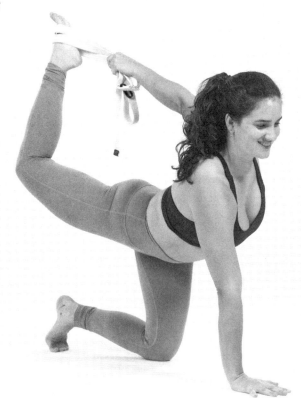

Ustrasana (Camel Pose)

Figure 8.43

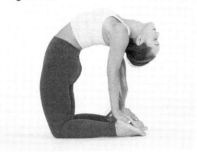

CHAIR VARIATIONS

Start off seated on a chair. Stand up and move around to the back of the chair, facing away from it and standing with the feet hip-width apart. Inhale and engage the muscles of the pelvic floor, draw the muscles of the lower abdomen in and up along the front of the body, lift the ribs away from the hips, engage the quadriceps and begin to send the pelvis forward to shift weight toward the front of the feet and open the front of the hips. Exhale and internally rotate the shoulders; reach back to hold the top of the backrest with the hands. Activate the muscles around the spinal axis and push the pelvis even farther forward (see fig. 8.44). Avoid overactivating the glutes. Only when the neck feels fully supported by the shoulders should an attempt be made to drop the head gently onto the pillow of the trapezius muscles and the gaze directed slightly upward. Stay for five breaths, then return to standing. This is a good option if getting up from and down to the floor is not advised in any capacity or if the knees are sore.

Figure 8.44

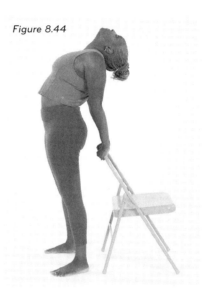

Start off seated on a chair. Slide the hips forward until the knees reach toward the floor. Settle the knees, shins, and feet on the floor, moving with sensitivity and awareness. If the knees are sore, consider placing a blanket under them. Allow the feet to gently root into the ground. Inhale and engage the muscles of the pelvic floor, draw the muscles of the lower abdomen in and up along the front body, lift the ribs away from the hips, engage the quadriceps, and begin to send the pelvis forward to shift weight toward the front of the feet and open the front of the hips. Exhale and internally rotate the shoulders; reach back to hold the lowest portion of the backrest with the hands. Activate the muscles around the spinal axis and push the pelvis even farther forward (see fig. 8.45). Only when the neck feels fully supported by the shoulders should an attempt be made to drop the head gently onto the pillow of the trapezius muscles and the gaze directed slightly upward. Explore a different hand and neck position. Slide the hands down along the legs of the chair and reach toward the feet or blocks near the feet. Once the hands are in contact with either the feet or a supportive object connected to the floor, bend into each of the joints of the spine and rest the head on the seat of the chair or a block on the seat of the chair (see fig. 8.46). It is always necessary to adjust the support for the size and shape of the body. Extend the neck and gaze toward the nose. Stay for five breaths, then return to sitting on the chair.

Figure 8.45

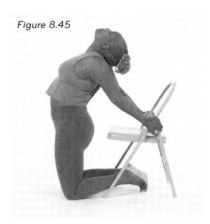

Figure 8.46

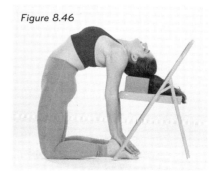

Figure 8.47

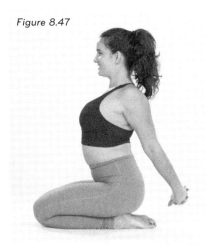

Figure 8.48

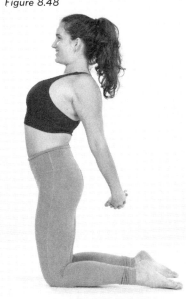

FLOOR VARIATION

Start off in Adho Mukha Svanasana. Exhale and come forward to a kneeling position by dropping the shins to the ground. Sit on the shinbones or immediately lift the hips, depending on the comfort of the knees. Align the knees, feet, and lower legs hip-width apart. Inhale and engage the muscles of the pelvic floor, draw the muscles of the lower abdomen in and up along the front body, lift the ribs away from the hips, engage the quadriceps, and begin to send the pelvis forward to shift weight toward the front of the feet and open the front of the hips. Extend the arms back behind the sacrum and interlock the fingers or hold a strap. Exhale and engage the back muscles; lift the sternum up and forward (see fig. 8.47). Inhale again and lift the pelvis off the lower legs, opening the front of the hips (see fig. 8.48). Gaze forward or toward the nose. Stay for five breaths, then exhale to move back into Chaturanga Dandasana and complete the vinyasa.

OTHER OPTIONS

Try the pose with two blocks. Place two blocks at their highest position on the floor on the outsides of the ankles. Exhale and internally rotate the shoulders, reach back and place the hands on the blocks, activate the muscles around the spinal axis, and push the pelvis even farther forward (see fig. 8.49). Only when the neck feels fully supported by the shoulders should an attempt be made to drop the head gently onto the pillow of the trapezius muscles. Once stable in the asana, gaze toward the nose or slightly upward (see figs. 8.50 and 8.51). Stay for five breaths, then exit the pose with the same level of integrity as was used to enter it. Inhale and lift the hands off the blocks; send the hips forward. Exhale and sink the hips back toward the feet. Inhale again and move back to Chaturanga Dandasana to complete the vinyasa.

Figure 8.49

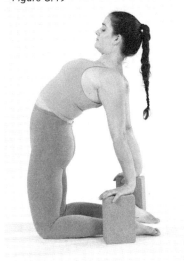

Figure 8.50

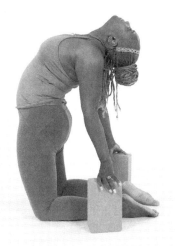

Figure 8.51

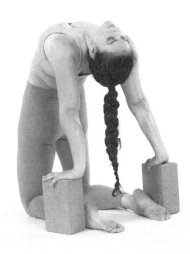

Laghuvajrasana (Little Thunderbolt Pose)

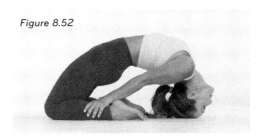

Figure 8.52

CHAIR VARIATION

Repeat the first option given for Ustrasana, while focusing on strengthening the legs, pelvic floor, and back muscles.

FLOOR VARIATION

Start off in Adho Mukha Svanasana. Exhale and come forward to a kneeling position by dropping the shinbones to the ground. Align the knees, feet, and lower legs hip-width apart. Stack two blocks behind the feet so they can support the head when the body shifts back. Inhale and engage the muscles of the pelvic floor, draw the muscles of the lower abdomen in and up along the front body, and lift the ribs away from the hips. Engage the quadriceps and begin to send the pelvis forward to shift weight toward the front of the feet and open the front of the hips. Internally rotate the shoulders; reach back and hold the ankles with the hands. Activate the muscles around the spinal axis, and firm the quadriceps even more. Once the trapezius muscles support the neck, allow the head to gently drop slightly back. Exhale and bend the knees even more to pitch the body back. Do not allow the pelvis to collapse and do not try to deepen the backbend. Instead, allow the body to travel more laterally backward along the horizontal plane to enter the pose. While moving back into the pose, keep the inner edges of the wrists snuggled in behind the inside edges of the heels and push down firmly (don't pull). Think about going long rather than folding, and focus on the stabilization elements of the pose. Keep going back until either the legs feel they cannot support the movement or the head rests on the blocks (see fig. 8.53). If the blocks and the mat feel too hard, try this variation with a bolster and blankets under the knees (see fig. 8.54). Gaze toward the nose. Stay here for five breaths. Inhale and lift the head off the blocks, send the hips forward, and return to the kneeling position. Exhale and sink the hips toward the feet. Inhale again and move back to Chaturanga Dandasana to complete the vinyasa.

Figure 8.53

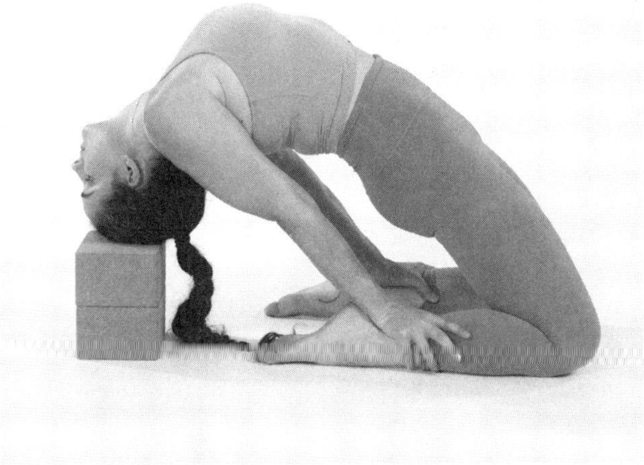

Figure 8.54

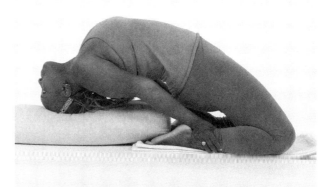

Figure 8.55

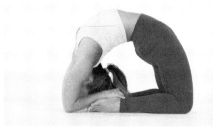

Figure 8.56

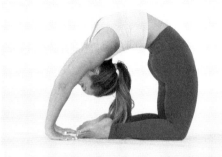

Kapotasana A and B (Pigeon Pose A and B)

This particular pose is considered to be extremely difficult and represents one of the greatest challenges of the Ashtanga Yoga practice. All students are advised to proceed slowly and perhaps consider staying at this asana for a few months, if not a few years, before proceeding. While it is not crucial that every student achieve the same level of physical aptitude in this asana, it is certainly recommended that each student utilize the pose to dive as deeply as possible into the inner lessons.

It should be noted that the Sanskrit word for pigeon is *kapotasana*. As Pigeon Pose has been popularized in the West mostly as an entirely different pose that focuses on opening the hips, it may be useful to understand the origin of this apparent confusion. There is an asana in the Third Series of Ashtanga Yoga called Eka Pada Raja Kapotasana. The leg position of this asana has been isolated and used for opening the hips. Throughout this text, whenever Pigeon Pose is recommended as a preparatory pose or an alternative option for another pose, it is called Kapotasana Variation or Pigeon Pose Variation for this purpose. If there is any doubt about which version of Pigeon Pose to practice, please consult the figures for greater clarification.

CHAIR VARIATION

Working deep backbends from the chair can feel both supportive and freeing. It may be useful for every practitioner to work on this option to better release and open the upper back. So often backbends remain localized in the lower back and fail to achieve the purpose of lifting the energy up from the base of the spine to the top of the head along the central channel.

Place an open-back chair near and facing away from a wall; place a bolster on the floor in front of the chair. Sit on the chair facing the wall and slide the feet through the open backrest. Press the soles of the feet firmly against the wall and align the legs hip-width or just slightly wider apart.

Figure 8.57

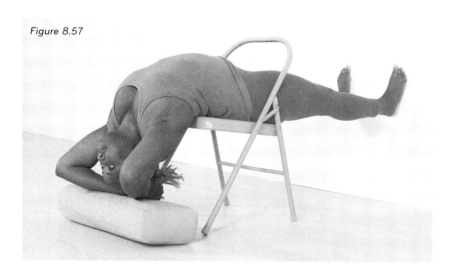

Engage the quadriceps and actively push into the wall to build a firm foundation in the legs. If a free wall isn't available, then place two blocks at their highest position on the floor to the outside of the ankles. Inhale and engage the muscles of the pelvic floor, draw the muscles of the lower abdomen in and up along the front of the body, lift the ribs away from the hips, and lower the body backward. Align the front edge of the seat of the chair with the lower ribs to support the upper spine and encourage spinal extension. Elongate the front of the body and open the front of the hips. Exhale and externally rotate the shoulders, reaching back with the hands toward the bolster; bend the elbows, interlace the fingers around the back of the head as in a headstand, and ground with the strength of the arms (see fig. 8.57). The head can make contact with the bolster or remain floating in the air, depending on the level of flexibility and comfort. Activate the muscles around the spinal axis, and push into the wall through the legs. Stay for five to ten breaths. Bend the knees, reach the feet down to the ground, and slide the hands up the sides of the chair to gently guide the torso back to an upright position to exit the pose.

FLOOR VARIATIONS

Start off in Adho Mukha Svanasana. Exhale and come forward to a kneeling position by dropping the shinbones to the ground. Align the knees, feet, and lower legs hip-width apart. Place the knees on a blanket or cushy mat. Place a bolster just behind the feet so it will support the head when the body shifts back. Inhale and engage the muscles of the pelvic floor, draw the muscles of the lower abdomen in and up along the front of the body, lift the ribs away from the hips, and engage the quadriceps. Exhale and send the pelvis forward to shift weight toward the front of the feet and open the front of the hips. Place the hands in the same position as in Laghuvajrasana and continue exhaling until the head touches the bolster. If this entry feels too difficult, try to lie down on the bolster from a kneeling position and then lift the hips to tuck the head back into the extended

Figure 8.58

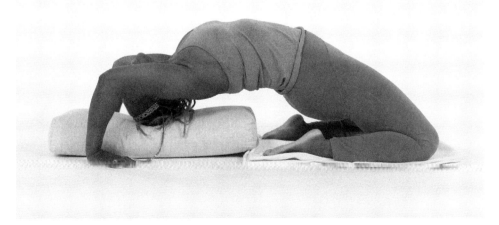

position. Allow as many breaths as necessary to enter the pose. Once the head rests on the bolster, gently lift the hands above the head and reach for the outsides of the bolster. Externally rotate the shoulders, place the palms on the floor along the outer edges of the bolster, and draw the elbows in line with the shoulders (see fig. 8.58). Activate the muscles around the spinal axis, and firm the quadriceps even more. Avoid overactivating the glutes. Gaze toward the nose. Stay here for five breaths. If the head feels supported, consider straightening the arms and lifting the head off the bolster for another five breaths. If the legs feel exhausted, then slide the torso back onto the bolster to exit the pose. If the legs are still strong, then inhale and lift the head off the bolster, send the hips forward, and return to the kneeling position. Exhale and sink the hips toward the feet. Inhale again and move back to Chaturanga Dandasana to complete the vinyasa.

OTHER OPTIONS

Try the pose with a yoga wheel. Start off in a kneeling position and align the knees, feet, and lower legs hip-width apart. Place the wheel between the feet so it will support the pelvis and back when the body shifts backward. Inhale and engage the muscles of the pelvic floor, draw the muscles of the lower abdomen in and up along the front of the body, lift the ribs away from the hips, and engage the quadriceps. Exhale and settle the pelvis, the torso, and the rest of the body on the wheel. Once the head rests comfortably on the floor or against the wheel, gently walk the hands along the head to eternally rotate the shoulders and clasp the edges of the wheel (see fig. 8.59). Activate the muscles around the spinal axis, and firm the quadriceps even more. Avoid overactivating the glutes. Gaze toward the nose. Stay here for five breaths. Inhale and release the wheel, send the hips toward the floor, and allow the wheel to lift the head and torso to return to the kneeling position with support. Exhale and settle. Inhale again and move back to Chaturanga Dandasana to complete the vinyasa.

Here is another way to work with Kapotasana. Start off in a kneeling position and align the knees, feet, and lower legs hip-width apart. Inhale and engage the muscles of the pelvic floor, draw the muscles of the lower abdo-

Figure 8.59

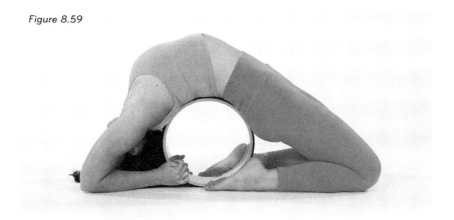

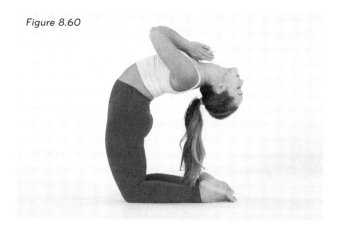

Figure 8.60

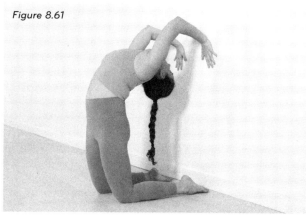

Figure 8.61

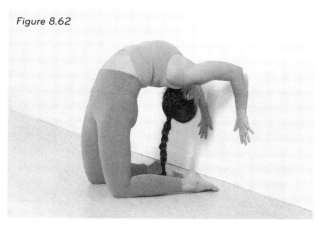

Figure 8.62

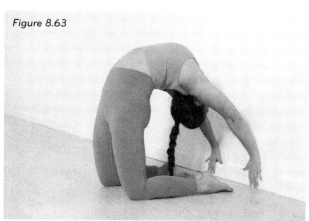

Figure 8.63

men in and up along the front of the body, lift the ribs away from the hips, engage the quadriceps, bring the hands into prayer position, and gently drop the head back (see fig. 8.60). Avoid overactivating the glutes. Stay here for five to fifteen breaths to create space. Return to the kneeling position.

This can also be done in front of a wall. Follow the preceding instructions facing away from the wall, but instead of returning to a kneeling position, exhale and extend the arms back toward the wall. Maintain the external rotation of the shoulders, and align the arms with them. Maximize the space between the ribs and the hips, send the pelvis forward, root down with the legs, and gaze between the hands (see fig. 8.61). If the body feels good, explore walking the hands down the wall. Avoid crunching the spine, overactivating the glutes, or forcing the body in any way (see fig.8.62). Stay for five breaths with bent elbows. Straighten the arms, engage the shoulders to facilitate a deep external rotation, send the pelvis farther forward, and engage the quadriceps and pelvic floor strongly (see fig. 8.63). Gaze toward the feet or the nose. Stay for five additional breaths, then walk gently back up the wall to exit the pose. Exhale and settle. Inhale again and move back to Chaturanga Dandasana to complete the vinyasa.

Figure 8.64

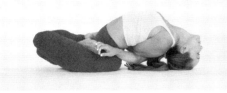

Figure 8.65

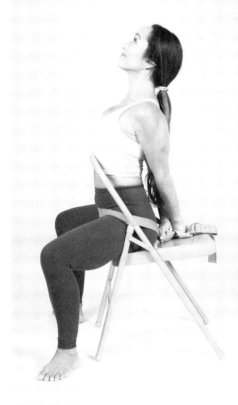

Supta Vajrasana (Reclining Thunderbolt Pose)

CHAIR VARIATION

Repeat one of the variations given for Ustrasana, following the movements of the vinyasa as appropriate for the body. Or try this alternative. Slide the legs under the backrest of the chair and externally rotate the hip joints. Thread a strap around the front of the body and cross the elbows behind the back. Hold the ends of the strap with the hands, internally rotate the shoulders, lift the chest, and gently gaze upward or toward the nose (see fig. 8.65). Stay for five breaths, then pulse up and down three times. Stay for an additional five breaths.

FLOOR VARIATION

If Padmasana is accessible but the hands are not yet ready to bind the lotus, use a strap. Sitting in Padmasana, engage the feet and wrap a strap around the insteps, placing the ends beside the hips. Cross the arms around the back, starting with the left arm first, and grasp the ends of the strap firmly. Inhale and engage the muscles of the pelvic floor, draw the muscles of the lower abdomen in and up along the front of the body, lift the ribs away from the hips, internally rotate the shoulders, and engage the back muscles. This asana is best practiced with a person or object like a solid piece of furniture supporting the knees, but that is not always readily available. Only with the support of an external object is it recommended to complete the full cycle of thirteen breaths. If practicing alone without any support, exhale and gently bend backward until the head touches either the floor or a bolster or until a comfortable limit is reached (see fig. 8.66). Hold for five breaths, gazing toward the nose. Inhale to come up. If Padmasana is not accessible, then fold the legs into a comfortable cross-legged position and wrap a strap around the pelvis to support the same movement (see fig. 8.67).

Figure 8.66

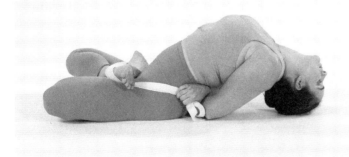

Figure 8.67

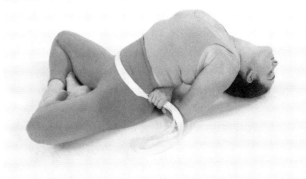

Bakasana (Crane Pose)

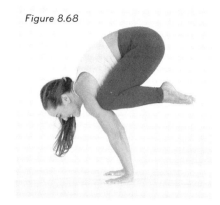

Figure 8.68

CHAIR VARIATION

A good alternative to Bakasana for the chair could be to repeat the practice of Utkatasana with the hands or elbows resting on the thighs, or try the option presented later in this chapter for Karandavasana (Himalayan Duck Pose).

FLOOR VARIATION

Start off in Adho Mukha Svanasana. Stack two blocks hip-width apart, a short distance behind the hands. Walk the feet forward and step onto the blocks. Bend the elbows, drawing them in to remain shoulder-width apart. Activate the core muscles of the shoulder girdle and the torso. Draw the lower ribs in toward the spine to maximize spinal and front-body compression. Tuck the tailbone, and engage the muscles of the lower abdomen and pelvic floor. Bring the thighs as close to the torso as possible; bend the knees and settle them on the upper edges of the triceps, as close to the armpits as possible. Gaze forward between the hands. Transfer weight onto the shoulders and feel the body weight gently moving into the stability of the upper body (see fig. 8.69). Stay for five breaths. If the shoulders have a hard time stabilizing, wrap a strap around the upper arms. With the additional support, it may feel safe to lift one foot off the blocks (see fig. 8.70). Do not be too quick to lift both feet off the blocks. Holding the foundation of the asana for many breaths helps build strength safely over time. Rushing to lift or jump the feet off the blocks may place too much pressure on the shoulders before they are ready to bear weight.

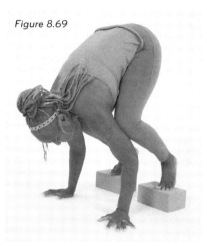

Figure 8.69

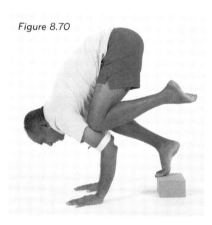

Figure 8.70

OTHER OPTIONS

Try this pose from a reclining position. Lie flat on the back. Extend the arms upward and point the palms toward the ceiling. Activate the core muscles of the shoulder girdle and torso. Draw the lower ribs in toward the spine to maximize spinal and front-body compression. Tuck the tailbone and engage the muscles of the lower abdomen and pelvic floor. Bring the thighs as close to the torso as possible; bend the knees and settle them on the upper edges of the triceps, as close to the armpits as possible (see fig. 8.71). Hold the floating position of Bakasana for five to ten breaths, then return to lying down. This is a great variation for those with sore or injured wrists. This can also be practiced on a large chair, sofa, or bed if getting up from and down to the floor is not advised.

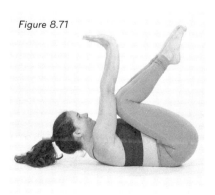

Figure 8.71

Figure 8.72

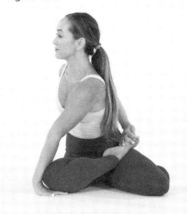

Bharadvajasana (Bharadvaja's Twist)

CHAIR VARIATION

Start off seated on a chair with the legs hip-width apart. Externally rotate the right hip joint, place the right foot on the lower edge of the left thigh just above the knee, and flex the right foot gently. Engage the muscles of the pelvic floor, and ground through the hips and legs to stabilize the pelvis. Inhale and lengthen the spine, draw the muscles of the lower abdomen in toward the spine, lift the ribs away from the hips, reach the right arm around the back toward the backrest of the chair, extend the left arm around the outer edge of the right thigh, and lift the sternum. Exhale to twist along the spinal axis while maintaining length and space throughout the body (see fig. 8.73). Do not pull on the backrest or on the body to force a twist. Instead, focus on the feeling of elongation, and gaze delicately over the right shoulder. Allow energy to flow up from the tip of the tailbone, through the central channel, and out from the top of the head. Stay for five breaths, then repeat on the other side. Return to seated.

Figure 8.73

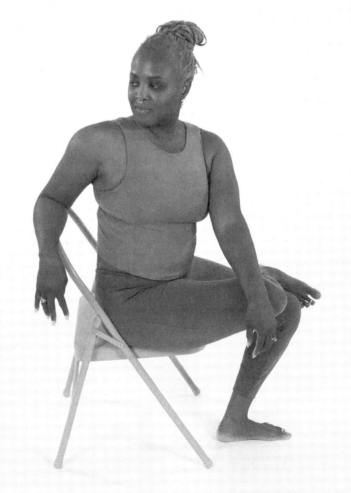

FLOOR VARIATION

Start off in Dandasana with a block behind the hips. Settle both sitting bones on the block. Internally rotate the left hip joint; fold the left leg back around the outer edge of the block so the shinbone rests on the floor and the left foot is pointed. Externally rotate the right hip joint so the right knee points out to the side, the shinbone folds under, and the sole of the foot nestles along the inner edge of the left thigh. Inhale to lengthen the spine, draw the ribs away from the hips, and create space along the chest and shoulders. Engage the muscles of the pelvic floor, and draw the muscles of the lower abdomen in toward the spine. Exhale and twist gently. Place the right hand behind the body and reach the fingertips toward the floor. Place the left hand along the right thigh, but avoid pulling or yanking on the leg to force the twist (see fig. 8.74). Maintain length and space between the vertebrae and around the chest and collarbone.

Keep the sitting bones and both sides of the pelvis grounded as part of the foundation of the twist. While the upper torso is twisting and lifting, the pelvis remains grounding and rooting. This counteraction is the essence of the pose. Check in with the right knee, and explore the possibility of folding the right leg up into half-lotus along the left hip crease. Continue the external rotation, closing the knee joint to facilitate this movement. Place a block under the right knee for additional support. Listen to the body; either exit the half-lotus and settle into the pose as previously instructed, or settle into the half-lotus and continue from here.

Once the half-lotus is firmly settled, reach the right arm around the back toward the right foot, and gently clasp the foot with a strap while pressing down lightly to ground the hips and shoulders (see fig. 8.75). If the body feels safe, explore removing the supportive block under the right knee and the strap. Stop immediately if there is any sharp pain or pressure around the right knee (see fig. 8.76). Stay for five breaths, then repeat on the other side. Return to seated.

Figure 8.74

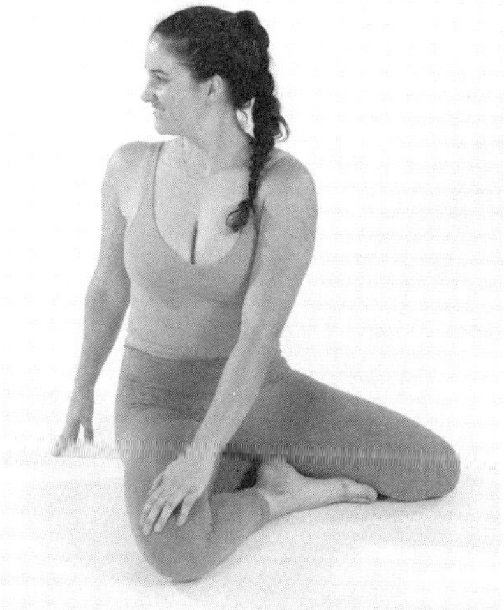

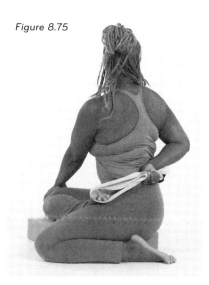

Figure 8.75

Figure 8.76

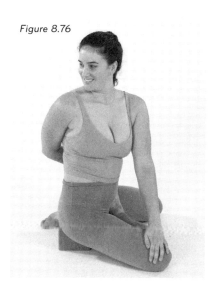

Figure 8.77

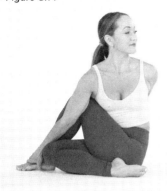

Ardha Matsyendrasana
(Half Lord of the Fishes Pose)

CHAIR VARIATION

Start off seated on a chair. Cross the right leg over the left. Stabilize the left leg and root it down into the ground. Inhale to create space. Exhale and gently twist to the right, placing the left hand on the right knee. Either extend the right arm open and out to twist to the right (see fig. 8.78), or place the right hand on the backrest of the chair and twist gently—do not pull (see fig. 8.79).

Feel free to substitute in any twisting action that works for the body. Another good option is to repeat the standing twist facing the chair given as a Chair Variation for Marichasana C in chapter 7. Stay for five breaths, then repeat on the other side. Return to seated.

FLOOR VARIATION

Start off in Dandasana. Fold the right leg over the left. Align the outer edge of the right foot with the outer edge of the left knee. Ground the left leg, press the left heel down, and firm the quadriceps. Engage the muscles of the pelvic floor, and draw the muscles of the lower abdomen in toward the spine to lift and support the spine and lower back. Avoid dumping weight into the lower back, and keep the torso snuggled close to the right hip. Twists are equal parts forward fold and twist, which can sometimes feel like contradictory movements for the body. Avoid twisting the pelvis or rotating around the sacroiliac joints. Inhale to lengthen the spine, lift the ribs away from the hips, and create space between the vertebrae, as well as the shoulders and the hips. Exhale and enter the twist to use the space that has been created. Draw the ribs in to fold around the spinal axis, move into hip flexion on the right side and allow the organs in the lower portion of the torso to feel a gentle pressure. Reach the right hand around the back, and press either the palm or the fingertips into the ground or a

Figure 8.78

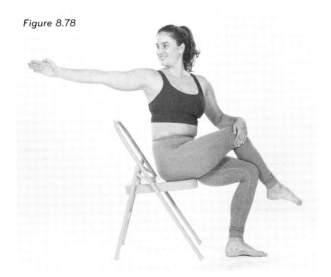

Figure 8.79

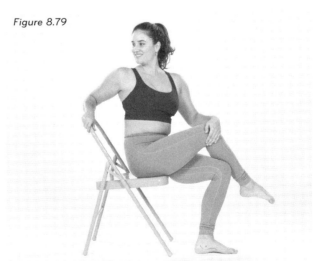

block. Fold the left arm around the outer edge of the right thigh. Bend the right elbow so the fingers point up. Firm the chest and shoulders to stabilize the upper limits of the twist (see fig. 8.80). If this feels comfortable, bend the left knee and fold the left leg so that the left toes point toward the back and the top of the left foot aims toward to the ground (see fig. 8.81). Gaze over the right shoulder. Stay for five breaths, then repeat on the other side. Return to seated.

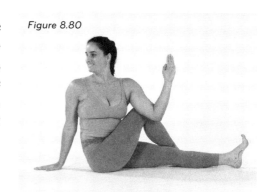

Figure 8.80

OTHER OPTIONS

Try the same pose with a block. Start off in Dandasana, and settle both sitting bones on a block. Externally rotate the left hip joint, and fold the left leg under the right. Align the left foot with the block, and point the left toes. Bend the right knee and internally rotate the right hip joint to cross the right leg over the left. Settle the right foot on the floor and align the outer edge of the right foot with the outer edge of the left knee. Engage the muscles of the pelvic floor, and draw the muscles of the lower abdomen in toward the spine to lift and support the spine and lower back. Avoid dumping weight into the lower back, and keep the torso snuggled close to the right hip. Avoid twisting the pelvis or rotating around the sacroiliac joints. Inhale to lengthen the spine, lift the ribs away from the hips, and create space between the vertebrae, as well as the shoulders and the hips. Exhale and enter the twist. Reach the right hand around the back, and press either the palm or the fingertips into the ground or a block. Fold the left arm around the outer edge of the right thigh. Bend the right elbow so the fingers point down and gently hold the right thigh. Firm the chest and shoulders to stabilize the upper limits of the twist and avoid twisting the collarbones (see fig. 8.82). Gaze over the right shoulder. Stay for five breaths, then repeat on the other side. Return to seated.

A reclining variation of Ardha Matsyendrasana can be a wonderful addition to the practice. Chair practitioners can try reclining options on a bed.

Figure 8.81

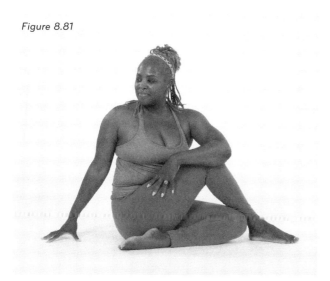

Figure 8.82

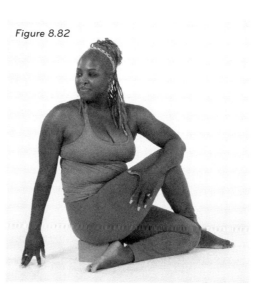

Figure 8.83

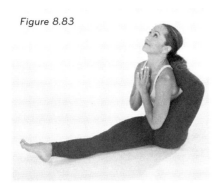

Figure 8.84

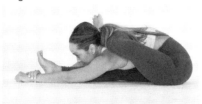

Figure 8.85

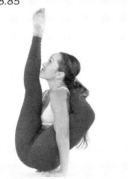

Eka Pada Sirsasana
(Foot behind the Head Pose)

With this asana, there are many variations and ways to work on the movement that will one day lead to putting the leg behind the head. What's most important is that the practice is a pathway that leads to deepening the sense of external hip rotation and the felt-sense of the body at the level of the hips. Explore these different options and find what works best for the practice and your body.

CHAIR VARIATION

Start off seated on a chair. Stand up and turn around to face the front of the chair. This variation can be considered a standing Kapotasana (Pigeon) Variation. Be sure the chair is stable and will not slide. If the chair isn't stable, then use a sofa or some other object with a solid base. Externally rotate the right hip joint and lift the right leg. Place the right lower leg along the seat of the chair. Engage the deep six hip rotator muscles to support the external rotation of the hip joint and stabilize the hips. Ground down through the left leg and engage the quadriceps. Activate the muscles of the pelvic floor, draw the muscles of the abdomen in toward the spine, draw the ribs away from the hips, and elongate the entire torso (see fig. 8.86). Place the hands on the hips, and equalize the pelvis to avoid hiking one hip higher than the other. Gaze forward. Stay for five breaths, then repeat on the other side. Return to seated.

Figure 8.86

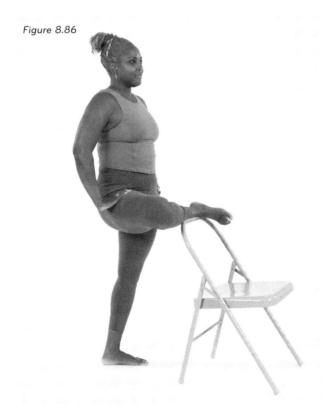

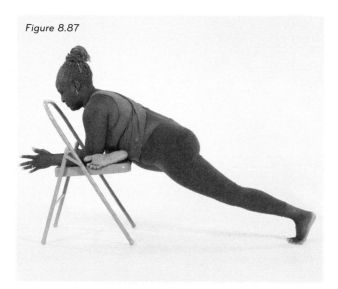

Figure 8.87

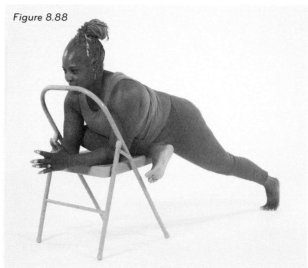

Figure 8.88

If the standing supported Kapotasana (Pigeon) Variation feels comfortable, try a different variation. Stand in front of the chair, facing the seat. Externally rotate the right hip joint and lift the right leg. Lay the outside of the lower leg along the middle of the seat and let the knee point out to the right side. Engage the deep six hip rotator muscles to support the external rotation of the hip joint and stabilize the hips. Ground down through the left leg and engage the quadriceps. Activate the muscles of the pelvic floor, draw the muscles of the abdomen in toward the spine, draw the ribs away from the hips, and elongate the entire torso (see figs. 8.87 and 8.88). Extend the left leg back until the leg is completely straight, curl the toes under, flex the foot, and maintain the stability of the left leg as the foundational support of the pose. Fold the chest forward and increase the hip flexion on the right side. Settle the hands or elbows on the seat of the chair just in front of the shinbone. Engage the shoulder girdle, and draw the lower ribs in toward the spine to stabilize the front body and support the torso. Gaze forward or toward the nose. Stay for five breaths, then repeat on the other side. Return to seated.

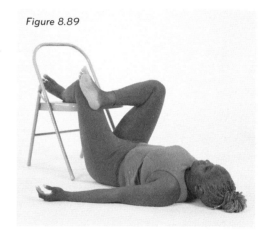

Figure 8.89

If balancing Kapotasana (Pigeon) Variation on the chair seems ill-advised or inaccessible, try to rest the leg that is externally rotating on a sofa or bed. If that still doesn't feel good, then try from a reclining position on a sofa or bed. When Kapotasana (Pigeon) Variation is practiced in a reclining position, it is sometimes referred to as Supta Kapotasana (Reclining Pigeon), and some options that might work on a sofa or bed are also shown in the next Floor Variations section. Lie on the back in front of a chair or lie down on a sofa or bed. Place both lower legs on the seat or lift both legs up. Externally rotate the right hip joint, place the right foot on top of the left knee, and open the right leg out to the side. Keep a slight engagement in the left leg for stability, and relax the right hip joint as much as possible. Let the emphasis in this variation be on relaxing and releasing the muscles around the deep six of the right hip, the lower back, and any areas of stress or tension in the body. Allow the hands to rest on the floor and close the eyes (see fig. 8.89). Keep a very light activation of the pelvic floor, or explore releasing the muscles of both the pelvic floor and the abdomen to enter a deeper state of relaxation.

FLOOR VARIATIONS

Kapotasana (Pigeon) Variation is a good alternative to the leg-behind-the-head movement. This works the necessary muscle group for external rotation of the hip joint and can be adapted to more bodies more easily. Starting off in Adho Mukha Svanasana, place a bolster and block on the mat. Place the bolster just in front of the hands, and keep the block over on the right side of the mat. Externally rotate the right hip joint and slide the right knee forward until it comes as close to the right hand as possible. Close the right knee joint and slide the block under the right hip. Engage the muscles of the pelvic floor, draw the muscles of the lower abdomen in toward the spine, and fold the lower ribs in toward each other. Align the pelvis to point symmetrically toward the ground, and avoid sliding the weight onto one hip. Keep the left leg extended back and begin to fold forward. Place the elbows on the bolster shoulder-width apart (see fig. 8.90). Eventually, it may feel good to fold all the way forward and rest on the bolster (see fig. 8.91). Gaze forward. Stay for five breaths, then repeat on the other side.

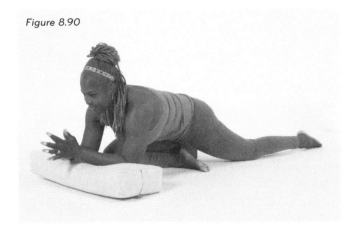

Figure 8.90

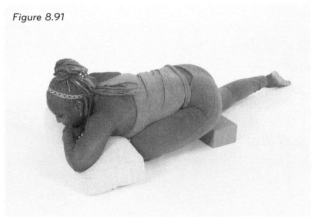

Figure 8.91

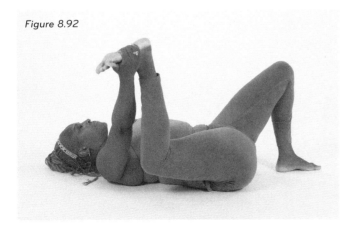

Figure 8.92

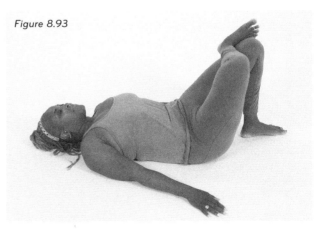

Figure 8.93

Another way to work the hyper hip flexion needed for this pose is from a half version of Ananda Balasana (Happy Baby Pose). Lie on the back. Bend both knees and align the feet just slightly wider than hip-width apart. Engage the muscles of the pelvic floor, draw the muscles of the lower abdomen in toward the spine, and fold the lower ribs in toward each other. Lift the right leg up toward the chest, point the sole of the foot up toward the ceiling, and hold the foot with the right hand. If holding the foot is not accessible, then hold anywhere along the right leg that works. Focus on deepening the hip crease and activating the deep six hip rotator muscles (see fig. 8.92). Do not pull forcefully with the right hand. Focus a bit more on the elements of release and relaxation, but do not lose the foundational stability of the pelvis. Avoid attempting to put the leg behind the head from here; focus more on the stretching sensation to build flexibility, release the back muscles, and support the spine. Sometimes attempting to put the leg behind the head in this pose can put undue pressure on the knee. Instead, to work on the external rotation from reclining, externally rotate the right hip joint, place the right foot on top of the left knee, and open the right leg out to the side. Keep a slight engagement in the left leg for stability,

Figure 8.94

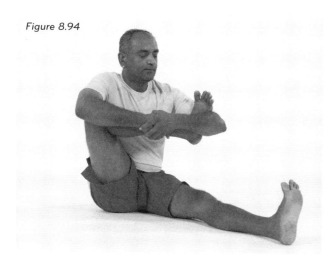

Figure 8.95

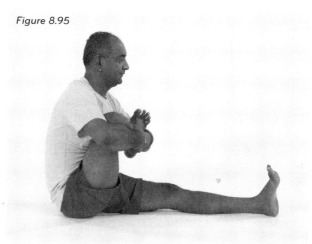

Figure 8.96

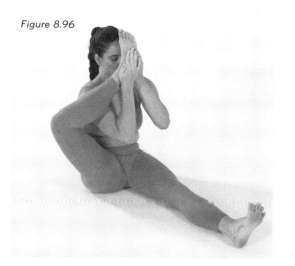

Figure 8.97

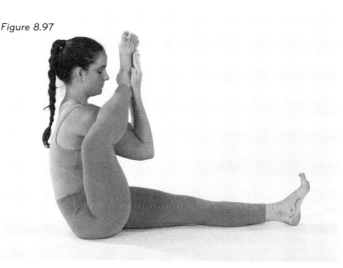

Figure 8.98

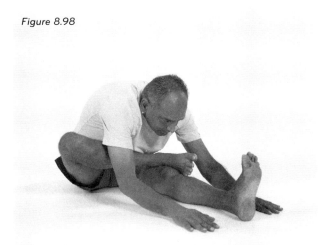

Figure 8.99

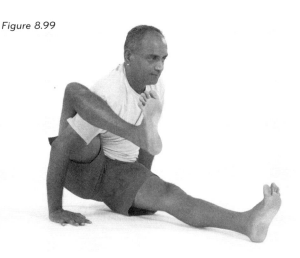

and relax the right hip joint as much as possible. Let the emphasis in this variation be on relaxing and releasing the muscles around the deep six of the right hip, the lower back, and any areas of stress or tension in the body. Allow the hands to rest on the floor and close the eyes (see fig. 8.93). Keep a very light activation of the pelvic floor, or explore releasing the muscles of both the pelvic floor and the abdomen to enter a deeper state of relaxation. Stay for five breaths, then repeat on the other side. Return to seated.

For another variation, start off in Dandasana. Externally rotate the right hip joint and lift the right leg. Bring the right shinbone up toward the chest; cradle the leg by wrapping the right arm around the right knee and placing the right foot in the elbow nook of the left arm. Engage the deep six hip rotator muscles to support the external rotation of the hip joint and stabilize the hips. Ground down through the left leg and engage the quadriceps. Activate the muscles of the pelvic floor, draw the muscles of the abdomen in toward the spine, draw the ribs away from the hips, and elongate the entire torso (see figs. 8.94 and 8.95). Gaze toward the nose or left toes. Think of this as a floor variation of Kapotasana (Pigeon) Variation.

If there is no pain in the right knee and a feeling of openness in the hip, it may be possible to explore a next step. Gently hold on to the right foot with both hands. Drop the right shoulder along the inside edge of the right calf muscle. Lift the right foot up toward the face while maintaining the stability of the torso. Avoid bringing the face down toward the foot; this may cause undue pressure to adversely impact the lower back. Stabilize the shoulders and collarbones while increasing the external rotation of the right hip joint (see figs. 8.96 and 8.97). Gaze at the nose or down. Stay for a few breaths and explore how the body wants to work. Feel free to explore the movement of putting the leg behind the head, but do not force or judge the body. Find the body's limit and respect that. Stay for at least five breaths in the variation that best supports the inner work of the practice.

Figure 8.100

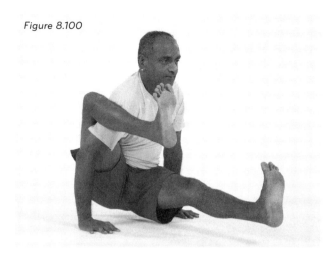

Figure 8.101

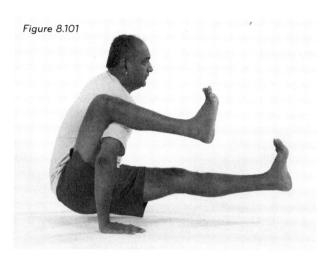

Exhale to fold forward while maintaining the shape of the legs. Either continue to support the right knee and shin along with the forward fold, or extend the arms forward along the sides of the left leg (see fig. 8.98). Gaze toward the nose or the left toes. Stay for five breaths. Inhale to return to seated.

It is also possible to replace the final lift of Eka Pada Sirsasana with Eka Hasta Bhujasana (Elephant Trunk Pose). Using a deep hyper hip flexion on the right side, slide the right leg behind the torso, point the right knee back, and bend the right knee around the upper edge of the right arm near the right shoulder. Curl the front body in and place the hands slightly in front of the hips and slightly wider than hip-width apart. Engage the core of the torso and the shoulder girdle firmly. Send the body weight forward and down into the foundation of the arms and upper body. Inhale and draw the pelvis back to lift the hips off the floor (see fig 8.99). Gaze forward or at the left toes. At first the left foot may remain on the floor; however, with consistent practice, strength builds and the left foot may float off the ground (see figs. 8.100 and 8.101). Do not kick or jump in an attempt to rush the process of building strength. Follow the technique and allow the body to find its own way into the pose. Stay for at least one full breath, then either jump back from here or return to seated. Find the way that works to flow through the vinyasa and then repeat on the other side. Note that one side of the body is likely tighter or more flexible than the other. Do not worry about achieving perfect symmetry. Practice with a subtle sensitivity to the sensations in the hip, and let that be the true goal of the practice.

Figure 8.102

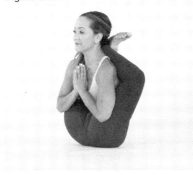

Figure 8.103

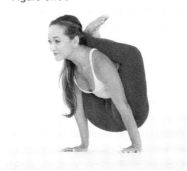

Dwi Pada Sirsasana
(Both Legs behind the Head Pose)

To adapt this asana to your practice, it may be useful to pause and reflect on the key elements that compose the pose and then choose to focus on what best supports the work you need to do in your practice. The key elements of Dwi Pada Sirsasana are external rotation of the hips, elongation of the back muscles to support a healthy spinal flexion, hyper hip flexion, stabilization of the shoulders, and balance. This might sound overwhelming, and truthfully, this pose often *is* overwhelming. Choosing one key element to focus on may help make the pose more accessible and less intimidating.

CHAIR VARIATION

To adapt Dwi Pada Sirsasana to a chair yoga practice, one idea is to repeat the same adaptation given for either Bujapidasana or Supta Kurmasana from the Primary Series in chapter 7. Lying on a bed or sofa and practicing Ananda Balasana as described for the next asana in the series, Yoganidrasana (Yogic Sleep Pose), is also a good option. Or it might be advisable to work the forward fold in a wide-legged position like Prasarita Padottanasana. These are just some of the options for adaptation. Continue to explore what works for the body and the practice.

Figure 8.104

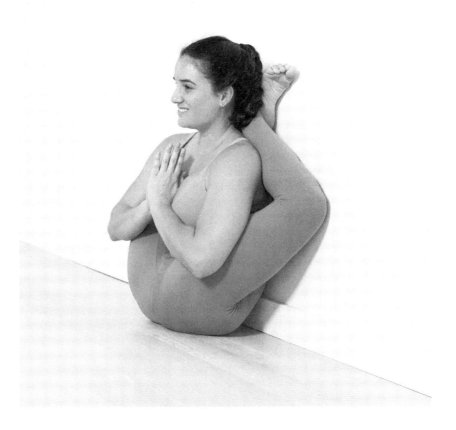

FLOOR VARIATION

Supporting the back can be key to making this asana accessible from the floor. Start off in Dandasana; a bolster behind the hips, or brace the hips against a wall. Gently curl the lower abdomen in, tuck the tailbone under, and engage the muscles of the pelvic floor. Externally rotate the left hip joint and lift the left leg up toward the chest, shoulder, and ear. Put the leg behind the head following the same instructions outlined for Eka Pada Sirsasana. Use the wall to support the back, and lift the head to actively push into the shinbone or ankle. Only when this leg feels stable and can support itself in the position should work proceed to put the second leg behind the head. Keep the left hand on the floor and avoid using it to try to hold the left leg in position. Externally rotate the right hip joint, bring the right leg around the right shoulder, and touch the feet together. Let the feet do the work of hooking around each other. If the feet are comfortably bound, then point the toes, and place the hands in the prayer position (see fig. 8.104). If the feet are struggling to maintain contact and there is undue pressure on the head, place the hands on the chin and push up; keep the feet hooked around each other and do not attempt to point the toes. Engage the deep six hip rotator muscles to support the external rotation of the hip joint and stabilize the hips. Bend the knees, ground down through the legs, and engage the quadriceps. Stabilize the collarbones, firm the chest, and push back into the legs with the strength of the shoulder girdle. Stay for five breaths.

Move away from the wall. Slide the calf muscles behind the upper arms and clasp the ankles (see fig. 8.105). If balance is accessible, bring the soles of the feet toward each other (see fig. 8.106). Lift up and complete the vinyasa in the same manner as for Supta Kurmasana in the Primary Series. As another alternative, try any of the options provided for Supta Kurmasana here as well.

Figure 8.105

Figure 8.106

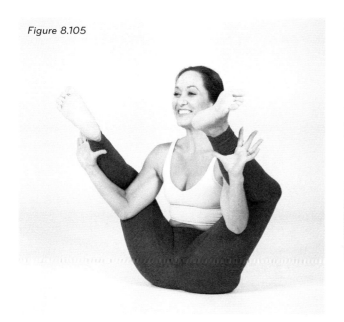
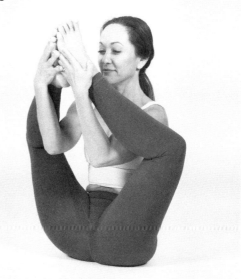

Figure 8.107

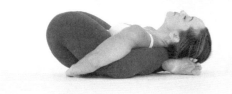

Figure 8.108

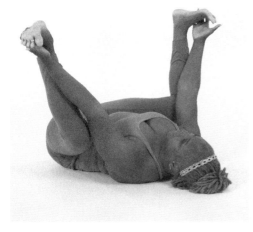

Figure 8.109

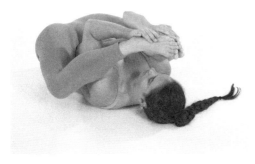

Figure 8.110

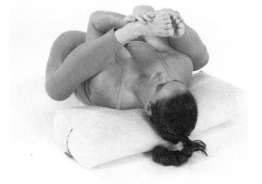

Yoganidrasana (Yogic Sleep Pose)

CHAIR VARIATION

To adapt Yoganidrasana to a chair yoga practice, follow the same suggestions outlined in the preceding pose and continue to explore new options that work best for external rotation of the hips from a reclining position.

FLOOR VARIATION

Try Ananda Balasana. Start off in Dandasana. Lie down on the back. Inhale and draw both legs into the chest. Lightly engage the muscles of the pelvic floor and draw the muscles of the lower abdomen in toward the spine, but do not tense the abdominal muscles. Move the feet and legs away from each other so the thighs slide around the outer edges of the torso. Reach the hands up along the inside or outside of the legs, and gently clasp the outside edges of the feet. Flex the feet and keep the soles pointing up (see fig. 8.108). If the hands do not comfortably reach the feet, then hold anywhere along the legs that feels comfortable, including the backs of the knees, the ankles, or wherever works to support the legs. Avoid pulling or forcing the legs. Instead, allow the weight of the arms to encourage increased hip flexion. The lower back rounds slightly, but do not lift the entire pelvis off the ground in an effort to deepen the pose. Keep the shoulders and head resting on the floor. Be sure the back feels safe and the bones of the spine are not pressing into the ground. Gaze toward the nose. Stay for five breaths.

OTHER OPTIONS

If this feels good, then add external rotation to Ananda Balasana to transform it more into something like a Floating Diamond Pose. Reach along the inside of the thighs and hold the outer edges of the ankles. Maintain the activation of the pelvic floor and the support of the muscles of the lower abdomen. Externally rotate the hip joints and point the knees out to the sides. Gently lift the sacrum off the ground and keep the head down to guide the feet closer to the face (see fig. 8.109). Do not compress the front body or try to lift the head up to the feet too much. If the back feels unsafe or could just use a little more support, place a bolster under the upper back and head (see fig. 8.110). Stay for five breaths. Gaze toward the nose.

Tittibhasana (Firefly Pose) A, B, C, and D

CHAIR VARIATION

To adapt Tittibhasana to a chair yoga practice, follow the same suggestions outlined for Dwi Pada Sirsasana, Supta Kurmasana, and Bujapidasana, and continue to explore new options that work best for hip flexion with straight and bent legs. It may be possible and fun to try entering the arm-balance portion of the pose with the assistance of the seat of a chair and two blocks. Sit on the chair and slide the hips slightly forward. Slide the torso between the thighs, and place the hands on the blocks. Reach the thighs around the upper arms and expand the chest. Engage the muscles of the pelvic floor, firm the shoulder girdle, and straighten the legs (see fig. 8.114). Stay for five breaths.

A *Figure 8.111*

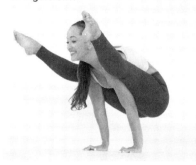

B & C (walking) *Figure 8.112*

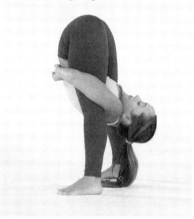

Figure 8.114

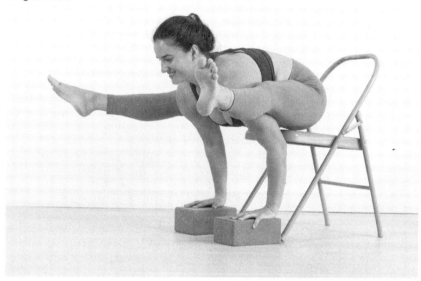

D *Figure 8.113*

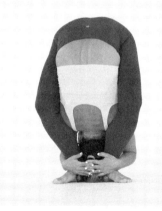

FLOOR VARIATION

When working the arm-balance portion of Tittibhasana A, the best way to make the pose more accessible is to bend the knees instead of straightening the legs. This allows the focus to remain on the hip flexion and bypasses hamstring flexibility, which can often be a big restriction. Any arm balance that relies deeply on flexibility is a dynamic flexibility pose and takes many years of practice to work through. Starting off in Adho Mukha Svanasana, inhale and walk the feet forward on the outsides of the hands. Allow the torso to slide between the thighs, bend the elbows, and settle the upper legs onto the shelf of the upper arms. Sink the hips back until the feet begin to lift. Straighten the legs as much as possible. Gaze toward the nose and stay for five breaths.

Use a strap to adapt for the next segments of Tittibhasana B, C, and D and make the asana more accessible. Start off standing with the feet

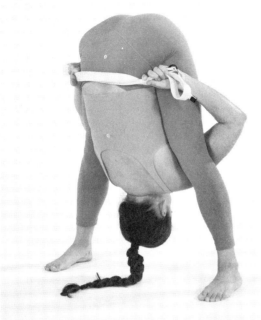

Figure 8.115

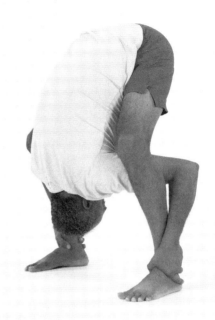

Figure 8.116

slightly wider than hip-width apart. Fold the torso between the thighs, bend the knees, maintain the activation of the pelvic floor and lower abdomen established in A position, and snuggle the shoulders under the knees. Hold a strap with one hand and lasso the strap around the lower back so both hands grip it firmly. Bend the elbows and internally rotate the shoulders. Stabilize the collarbones and the shoulder girdle to support the weight of the legs bearing down on the upper body. Tuck the head in toward the chest and gaze at the nose (see fig. 8.115). Stay for five breaths.

Maintain the same grip on the strap and proceed to Tittibhasana C. This portion of the pose is called "walking." Inhale and step the right foot forward. Exhale and step the left foot forward. Walk forward for a count of five, then walk backward for a count of five. Proceed immediately to Tittibhasana D.

Release the strap, keep the elbows bent, and wrap the hands around the ankles. Hold the ankles and straighten the legs as much as possible (see fig. 8.116). It is possible to lasso the strap around the ankles here if that feels more stable. Stay for five breaths. Then proceed immediately back to Tittibhasana A for at least one breath. Jump or step back to Chaturanga Dandasana and complete the vinyasa.

Note that Tittibhasana is a challenging dynamic flexibility, strength, and endurance pose. It is not easy, nor is it meant to be. The thighs may burn repeatedly. This is not an indication that something is wrong. When the thighs burn but the joints remain safe, this is evidence that the pose is working. Continue to explore different options that make the work of the pose more accessible.

Pincha Mayurasana
(Feathered Peacock Pose/Forearm Balance)

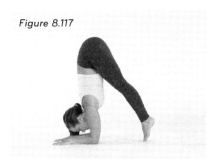
Figure 8.117

CHAIR VARIATION

If getting up from and down to the floor is not accessible, find ways to work on forearm strength from a seated position on a chair. Hold a block with both hands shoulder-width apart. Bend the elbows and lift the block up to head height, holding the elbows at the same height as the chest. Draw the elbows in to keep them in line with the shoulders. Activate the muscles of the pelvic floor, firm the abdomen, and draw the lower ribs in toward the spine (see fig. 8.119). Gaze forward or toward the nose. Stay for five breaths, then return to seated.

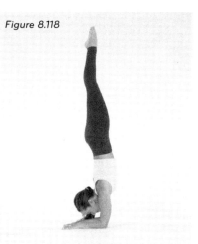
Figure 8.118

Try Makara Adho Mukha Svanasana (Dolphin Plank Pose) on the seat of the chair to build strength. Stand in front of the chair, bend the elbows, and align the forearms shoulder-width apart on the seat. Gently step back until the body is in a plank (see fig. 8.120). Maintain firm activation of the pelvic floor, the muscles of the abdomen, the shoulder girdle, and the legs. Gaze between the forearms at the seat of the chair. Stay for five breaths.

Try this with the chair against a wall for support. Stand up and move the chair against but facing away from the wall so the back legs of the chair rest on the floor just in front of the wall. Be sure the chair is stable and

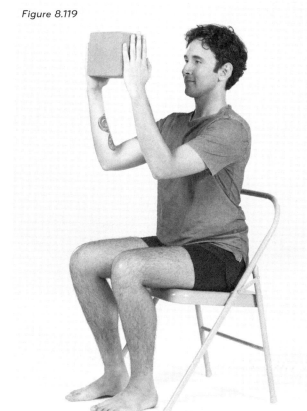
Figure 8.119

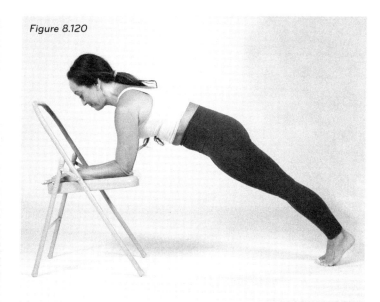
Figure 8.120

Figure 8.121

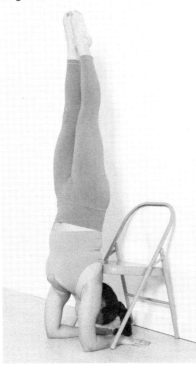

will not slide. Start off on hands and knees in front of the chair. Bend the elbows and slide the hands under and between the legs of the chair. Allow the forearms to be supported by the two front legs of the chair. Engage the muscles of the pelvic floor, firm the abdomen, and stabilize and strengthen the shoulders and chest. Walk the legs in as far as feels comfortable. Stay for a few breaths in Ardha Pincha Mayurasana (sometimes also known as Makarasana/Dolphin Pose) for the preparation.

If the body and breath feel stable, inhale and kick up to the wall. Slowly move the legs away from the wall and use the chair to help stabilize the upper back and find the center line. Gaze down toward the floor between the forearms (see fig. 8.121). Stay for five breaths, then return to Ardha Pincha Mayurasana.

FLOOR VARIATION

The best way to build strength for Pinchamayurasana is to work on the preparation for a long time. I do not recommend using a strap around the elbows because people usually push into the strap. This pushing outward is counterproductive and works against the healthy dynamics of pose. Instead, try the foundational preparatory poses and do not worry about forcing the body to go upside down before it's ready.

Start off in Adho Mukha Svanasana. Come down onto the knees. Bend the elbows and place them on the floor in line with the shoulders. Straighten the legs back. Engage the muscles of the pelvic floor, firm the abdomen, and stabilize and strengthen the shoulders and chest (see fig. 8.122). Stay for at least five breaths. Walk the legs in as far as feels comfortable and pivot forward toward the tips of the toes (see fig. 8.123). Stay for at least five breaths. Then either come down, explore lifting one leg, or come down and jump or step back to Chaturanga Dandasana to complete the vinyasa.

Figure 8.122

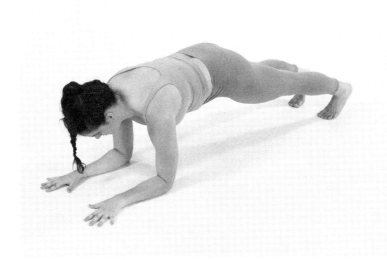

Figure 8.123

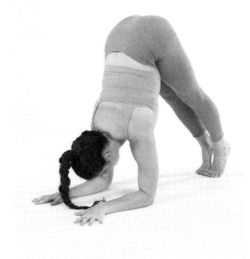

Karandavasana (Himalayan Duck Pose)

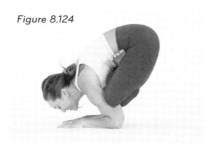
Figure 8.124

CHAIR VARIATION

Repeat the first instructions for Pinchamayurasana to work on the strength of the shoulders in the bent-elbow position. Keep holding the block and fold the torso forward. Draw the thighs and elbows gently inward, and touch the lower backs of the triceps to the knees (see fig. 8.126). Stay for five breaths. Gaze toward the nose. Do not attempt to fold the legs down from the chair-supported variation outlined previously.

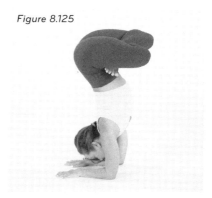
Figure 8.125

FLOOR VARIATION

The biggest challenge presented by Karandavasana for students with the strength to balance in Pinchamayurasana is folding into Padmasana while upside down. I have outlined various ways to work on the lotus position in *The Power of Ashtanga Yoga II*. Those instructions will not be repeated here. Instead, the variations for this pose focus on providing alternatives for students to whom the lotus position is inadvisable or inaccessible.

OTHER OPTIONS

To work on Karandavasana without the lotus position, merge the work of Bakasana with that of Pinchamayurasana. Instead of folding the legs into full lotus, bend the knees into the chest, and work toward Bala Kakasana (Baby Crow Pose) (see fig. 8.127). It may be useful to practice the pose itself from Ardha Pincha Mayurasana (Dolphin Pose) before lowering into it from Pinchamayurasana. Then, only when the pose itself feels stable, explore lowering onto the shelf of the triceps and lifting back up to balance. This adjustment of the pose does not decrease the demanding strength work required, but it does make the work of this difficult pose accessible for more students.

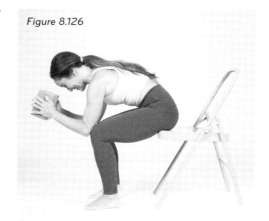
Figure 8.126

To do Bala Kakasana, activate the muscles of the pelvic floor, curl the spine into a deep spinal flexion, draw the lower ribs in, engage the muscles of the abdomen, firm the shoulders, draw the elbows in, and bend the knees onto the triceps as close to the armpits as possible. Gaze down to a single point between the hands. Stay for five breaths, then either return to Ardha Pincha Mayurasana (Dolphin Pose) or lift up, depending on what feels accessible to the body.

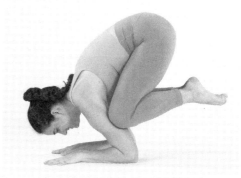
Figure 8.127

Figure 8.128

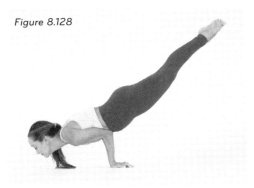

Mayurasana (Peacock Pose)

CHAIR VARIATION

For individuals who have a strong upper body but cannot get up from and down to the floor due to a restriction in the hips or knees, working on Mayurasana from standing may be a fun option. Use the backrest of a chair or a small stool in place of the blocks and work the lift following the same instructions detailed for the Floor Variation (see fig. 8.129).

FLOOR VARIATION

Figure 8.129

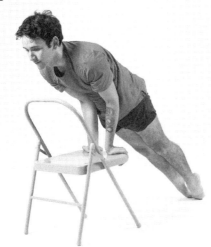

Try using two blocks. Start off on the hands and knees. Place the blocks in a rectangular formation spaced apart by about the same width as between the hips and the chest. Gently grip the block closest to the pelvis with both hands, with the fingers pointing out and the palms flattened on the center of the block. Engage the muscles of the pelvic floor, draw the muscles of the lower abdomen in toward the spine, firm the chest and shoulders, bend the elbows in toward each other, and settle the body onto the shelf of the elbows and triceps. Once the elbows make contact with the body, start to lean forward and transfer weight onto the arms. Pitch the head, chest, and shoulders forward and down until the forehead rests on the second block. Inhale and lift the legs back and up.

Explore different leg positions to make the lift more accessible. Try bending the knees in Baddha Konasana to keep the weight of the legs closer to the central axis (see fig. 8.130). Explore straightening the legs to increase the load and build more strength (see fig. 8.131). If the lift feels

Figure 8.130

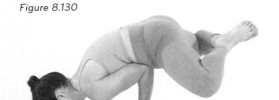

Figure 8.131

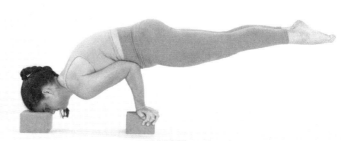

Figure 8.132

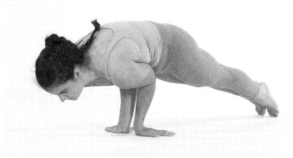

impossible, hold the prepare position with or without the blocks for a few breaths and feel strength building (see fig. 8.132). To get the feeling of the legs lifting off the ground, try placing a third block or bolster under the feet (see fig. 8.133). Avoid kicking to try to lift the legs off the ground. Instead, focus on the steady accumulation of strength in the muscles over many years of practice. Stay at what works for at least five breaths, then follow whichever variation of the vinyasa works best to continue the practice.

OTHER OPTIONS

With a wrist injury, it may be advisable to avoid bearing weight on the wrists entirely. In this case, Mayurasana can be inverted in much the same manner as Bakasana (see fig. 8.134). Continue to explore options that best support the work of the asana.

Figure 8.133

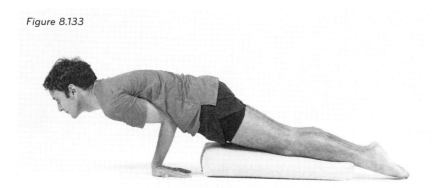

Figure 8.134

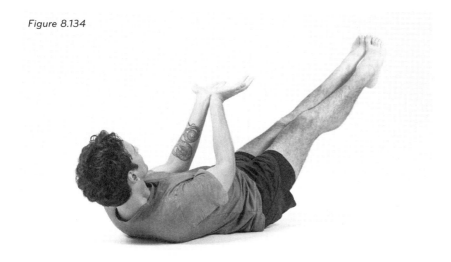

Figure 8.135

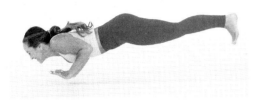

Nakrasana (Crocodile Pose)

Any variation of Kumbhakasana (Plank Pose) or Chaturanga Dandasana can be used as an alternative or adaptation to this pose. Depending on what restrictions are present and what areas can work, there is an infinite number of ways to practice the foundational elements of Nakrasana. Think about building up the strength for a good Kumbhakasana or Chaturanga Dandasana and then challenging that strength by lifting the arms or legs, eventually jumping or floating either the arms or legs or both for a moment, depending on which option is best for your body.

CHAIR VARIATION

Stand up and move around to the back of the chair. Use the backrest as a substitute for the floor. Place the hands on the backrest, shoulder-width apart, and straighten the arms. Step back from the chair to form a plank position with the body. Keep the feet close together. Stabilize the upper body, activate the pelvic floor, draw the muscles of the abdomen in toward the spine, and engage the legs (see fig. 8.136). Hold for at least five breaths to stabilize. Exhale and bend the elbows to enter a chair-supported Chaturanga Dandasana (see fig. 8.137). Inhale and straighten the arms. Repeat ten times. Do not attempt to jump or float the arms. Instead, work on the chair-supported push-up to build strength and stability.

FLOOR VARIATION

Kumbhakasana in all its variations is the best alternative to Nakrasana. If the wrists are sore, try Makara Adho Mukha Svanasana. If the shoulders are not yet strong enough, try Kumbhakasana with the knees down. If Kumbhakasana is solid, try the jumping movement directly from the traditional Kumbhakasana . If jumping the pose seems inaccessible, replace the jumping movement with ten push-ups from any variation of Kumbhakasana that works.

Figure 8.136

Figure 8.137

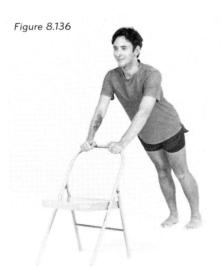

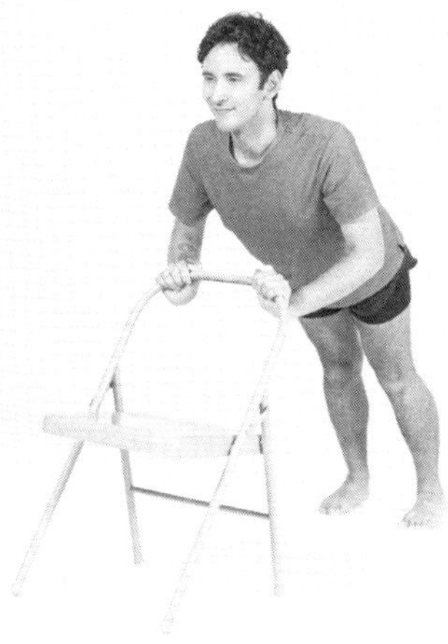

Vatayanasana (Horse Face Pose)

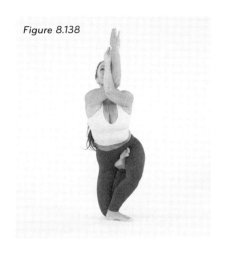

Figure 8.138

CHAIR VARIATION

Start off seated on a chair. Place the feet hip-width apart, and slide the sitting bones forward to the middle of the chair seat. Pivot slightly forward into the hip joints. Engage the muscles of the pelvic floor, draw the muscles of the lower abdomen in toward the spine, firm the quadriceps, and lengthen the spine by drawing the ribs away from the hips. Thread the arms together starting at the elbows. Place the right arm on top and fold the forearms around each other until the palms of the hands are close together (see fig. 8.139). Gently draw the arms in along the center line and lift up. Keep the shoulder blades rooted down the back. Gaze up toward the fingers. Stay for five breaths, then repeat on the other side. Return to seated.

Explore different leg positions. Try threading the legs as in Garudasana (Eagle Pose; see fig. 8.140) or stepping one leg back under the backrest of the chair (see fig. 8.141) and alternating legs when the arms switch.

FLOOR VARIATION

The adaptation for this pose removes the half-lotus and targets balance and shoulder flexibility without the strain of externally rotating the hips. Start off in Adho Mukha Svanasana. Step forward with the left foot. Turn the left foot out in a gentle external rotation. Drop the right knee in a kneel-

Figure 8.139

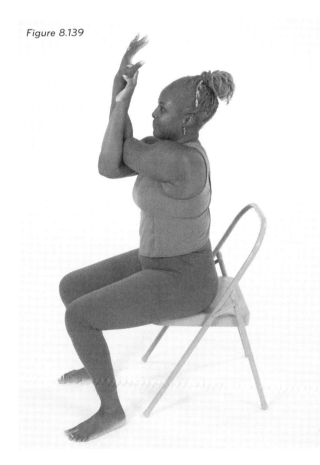

Figure 8.140

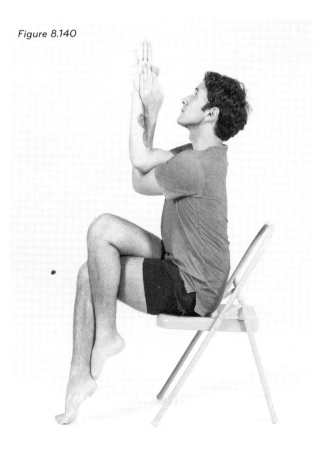

Figure 8.141

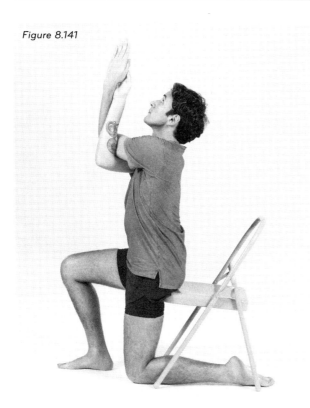

Figure 8.142

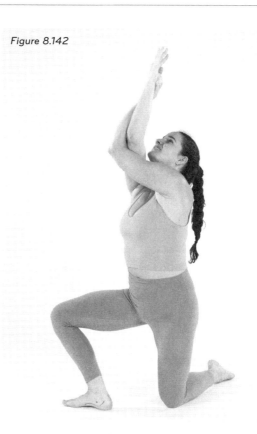

ing position. Sometimes this adaptation can feel like a knightly pose that brings up feelings of the Arthurian legends. Thread the arms together starting at the elbows. Place the right arm on top and fold the forearms around each other until the palms of the hands are close together (see fig. 8.142). Gently draw the arms in along the center line and lift up. Keep the shoulder blades rooted down the back. Gaze up toward the fingers. Stay for five breaths, then repeat on the other side, following the traditional vinyasa to return all the way to Samasthitih and continue with the practice.

Parighasana (Gate Pose)

Figure 8.143

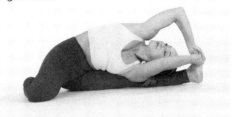

CHAIR VARIATION

Start off seated in a chair. Turn the whole body to the right. Bend the left knee and plant the left foot firmly on the floor. Allow a gently internal rotation of the left hip joint. Externally rotate the right hip joint and extend the right leg out to the side, at approximately a ninety-degree angle from the left leg. Flex the right foot, root the right heel down firmly, and engage the quadriceps. Inhale and engage the muscles of the pelvic floor, draw the muscles of the abdomen in toward the spine, lift the ribs away from the hips, and reach the left arm up by rotating the left shoulder externally. Exhale and reach the right arm down along the right leg, allowing a lateral stretch of the torso to facilitate a side bend (see fig. 8.144). Gaze up toward the left fingers. Stay for five breaths, then repeat on the other side. Return to seated.

Figure 8.144

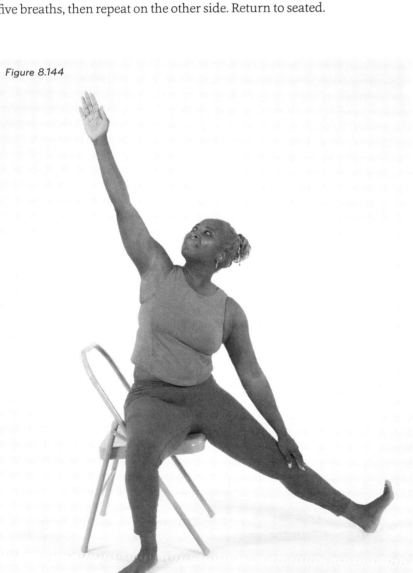

Figure 8.145

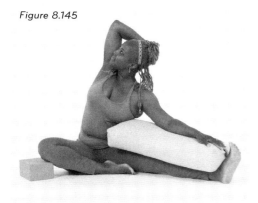

FLOOR VARIATION

Start off in Dandasana. Change the internal rotation in the right hip joint to external rotation and bend the right knee out to the side. Support the right knee with a block. Externally rotate the left hip joint and extend the left leg out; keep it straight. Place a bolster along the top of the left thigh. Inhale and engage the muscles of the pelvic floor, draw the muscles of the abdomen in toward the spine, and create space between the ribs and the hips. Exhale and fold the body to the left. Reach the left hand along the bolster toward the left foot, and lift the right arm to externally rotate the right shoulder. Gaze gently upward and slightly to the right (see fig. 8.145). Stay for five breaths, then repeat on the other side. Return to seated.

Next, elevate the hips to protect the knee and support the internal rotation of the hip joint. Sit on a block. Fold the right knee back, place the right foot along the outer edge of the block, and internally rotate the right hip joint. Externally rotate the left hip joint and extend the left leg out; keep it straight. Inhale and engage the muscles of the pelvic floor, draw the muscles of the abdomen in toward the spine, and create space between the ribs and the hips. Exhale and fold the body laterally. Reach the left hand along the inside edge of the left leg toward the left foot, and lift the right arm to externally rotate the right shoulder. Think about an open twist and lift the chest away from the left leg. Gaze gently upward and slightly to the right (see fig. 8.146). If the support of the block is not sufficient to alleviate any pain in the knee, then give the knee even more space by elevating the body off the block for an open variation of Parighasana (see fig. 8.147). Stay for five breaths, then repeat on the other side. Return to seated.

Figure 8.146

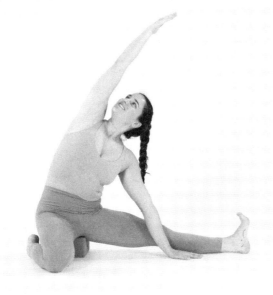

Figure 8.147

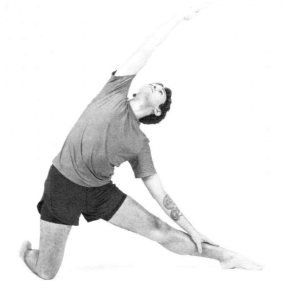

Gomukhasana (Cow Face Pose)

Figure 8.148   Figure 8.149

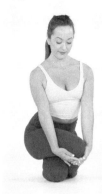
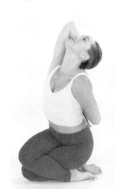

CHAIR VARIATION

Start off seated on a chair. Stabilize the left leg, and cross the right leg over the left. Rest the right foot on a block for added stability and ground down through both legs. Lean slightly forward to gently flex the hips, and wrap the hands around the right knee. Inhale and engage the muscles of the pelvic floor, draw the muscles of the abdomen in toward the spine, and create space between the ribs and the hips. Exhale and draw the shoulder blades down the back to delicately pull the body forward to a subtle spinal extension (see fig. 8.150). Gaze down. Stay for five breaths.

Hold a strap with the right hand and lift the right arm. Externally rotate the right shoulder, and bend the right knee. Internally rotate the left shoulder and reach the left hand around the back to clasp the strap. Lift the center of the chest and create more space between the ribs and the hips (see figs. 8.151 and 8.152). Gaze up gently. Stay for five breaths, then repeat on the other side. Return to seated.

Figure 8.150

Figure 8.151

Figure 8.152

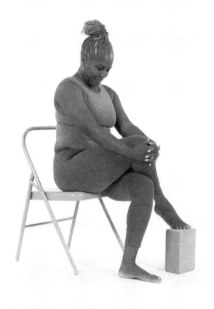
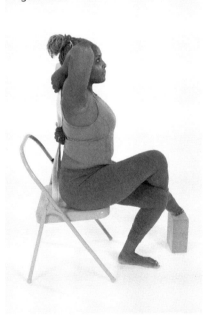
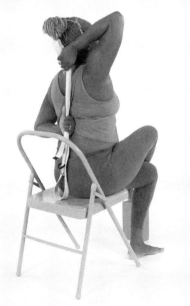

FLOOR VARIATION

Sit on a block or bolster to elevate the hips. Fold the legs on top of one another, with the thighs as close together as possible and following the center line of the body. Align the knees with the pubic bone and the center of the chest. Place the right leg on top, and externally rotate and close both hip joints. Lean slightly forward and wrap the hands around the right knee. Inhale and engage the muscles of the pelvic floor, draw the muscles of the abdomen in toward the spine, and create space between the ribs and the hips. Exhale and draw the shoulder blades down the back to del-

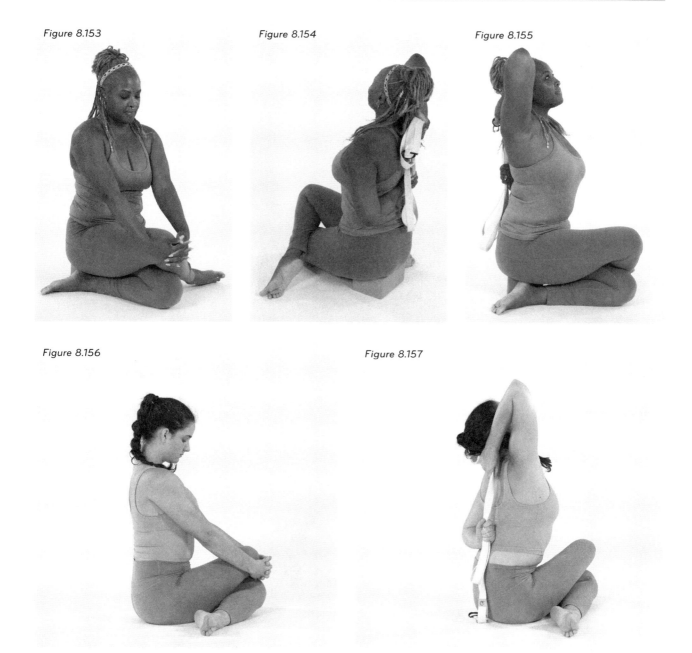

Figure 8.153

Figure 8.154

Figure 8.155

Figure 8.156

Figure 8.157

icately pull the body forward to a subtle spinal extension (see fig.8.153). Gaze down. Stay for five breaths.

Hold a strap with the right hand and lift the right arm. Externally rotate the right shoulder, and bend the right knee. Internally rotate the left shoulder and reach the left hand around the back and to clasp the strap. Lift the center of the chest and create more space between the ribs and the hips (see figs. 8.154 and 8.155). Gaze gently up. Stay for five breaths, then repeat on the other side. Return to seated.

If the knees feel safe, then try this without the block. Follow the instructions but sit directly on the floor (see figs. 8.156 and 8.157).

Supta Urdhva Pada Vajrasana
(Reclining Upward-Leg Thunderbolt Pose)

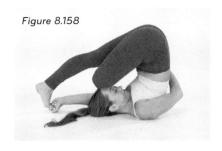

Figure 8.158

CHAIR VARIATION

To practice this asana from a chair, it is advisable not to attempt the rolling vinyasa. Instead, repeat the same instructions given for Bharadvajasana. If it feels comfortable, narrow the distance between the knees. If not, then repeat Bharadvajasana in a way that best supports the practice.

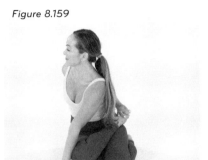

Figure 8.159

FLOOR VARIATION

If Bharadvajasana is comfortable, then it may be advisable and even fun to attempt the rolling entry into this asana. To make it more accessible, try wrapping a strap around the half-lotus foot instead of binding that foot with the hand (see fig. 8.160). Lie down, engage the muscles of the pelvic floor, and draw the muscles of the abdomen in toward the spine. Inhale and lift both legs over the head. Fold the right leg into half-lotus by externally rotating the hip joint and bringing the right foot toward the left hip crease. Place a strap around the right foot, and reach the left hand around the back to clasp the strap. Stay here for one breath.

Inhale and roll up. Fold the left leg under and into internal rotation as the body rolls up. Exhale and twist the torso to the right to enter the pose. Extend the left arm around the outer edge of the right knee. Keep the left hand lifted to give the body more space (see fig. 8.161). Stay for five breaths, then repeat on the other side. Return to seated.

Figure 8.160

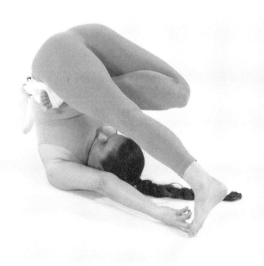

Figure 8.161

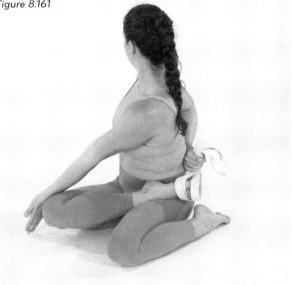

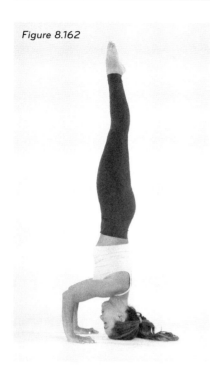

Figure 8.162

Mukta Hasta Sirsasana A
(Unsupported Headstand A/Tripod Headstand)

These three headstands are considered the "unsupported headstands." The hand support is placed away from the center line of the body so the neck has less support. Accordingly, those with tighter shoulders may find these hand positions more accessible. Proceed with caution, and do not force the body to invert or undue pressure may be placed on the neck. Any deviation from the center line in the cervical spine while inverting can lead to less-than-ideal results. Focus on the foundational strength and distribute the work of the asanas throughout the entire body. If at any time there is a crashing or crunching sensation in the neck, exit the pose immediately. Although difficult, these asanas are nevertheless safe to practice and immensely beneficial. Proceed with safety measures in place and the journey will be fruitful.

CHAIR VARIATION

Start off seated in a chair. Stabilize the core of the body to feel the center line. Engage the pelvic floor, draw the muscles of the lower abdomen and the rib cage in toward the spine, and reach up and out through the top of the head. Draw the shoulder blades down the back and relax the neck. Inhale to lift the arms, bend the elbows, and prepare the arm positions for the Tripod variation in this series of headstands. Either stay seated or stand up and work the alignment and shoulder strength of the pose without inverting (see fig. 8.163). Gaze toward the nose. Stay for five breaths, then return to seated. Between each of the headstands, flow through the vinyasa before proceeding to the next variation.

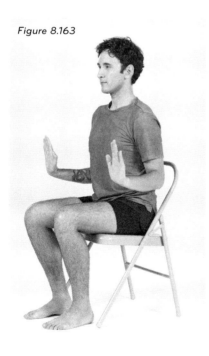

Figure 8.163

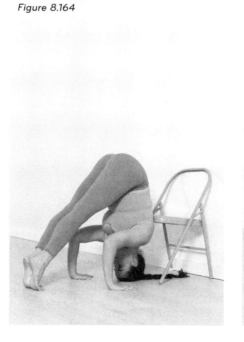

Figure 8.164

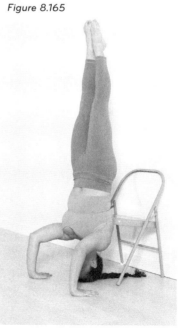

Figure 8.165

Try using a chair as support for the back and neck. Place a chair against a wall with the backrest facing the wall. Make sure the chair is secure and won't slide. Start on the hands and knees facing the chair and the wall. Engage the muscles of the pelvic floor, draw the muscles of the abdomen in toward the spine, draw the shoulder blades down the back, and stabilize the shoulder girdle and chest. Bend the knees and arms, and place the head on the floor just in front of the seat of the chair, almost in line with its front feet. Press the back against the seat of the chair. Inhale, straighten the legs up, and walk in to the tripod shape (see fig. 8.164). If the body is not yet ready to invert fully, then stay here and work the foundation of the prepare position. When the inversion feels accessible, inhale again and lift the legs to the center line of the body and find the balance (see fig. 8.165). Do not jump. If the balance is challenged, bend one knee and lightly touch the wall. Do not place both feet against the wall or the torso will deviate from the center line. Stay for five breaths, then return to the prepare position and come all the way down.

FLOOR VARIATION

Start off on the hands and knees. Engage the muscles of the pelvic floor, draw the muscles of the abdomen in toward the spine, draw the shoulder blades down the back, and stabilize the shoulder girdle and chest. Bend the knees and arms, and place the head on the floor to form the tripod shape. Inhale, straighten the legs up, and walk in to the prepare position (see fig. 8.166). If the body is not yet ready to fully invert, then stay here and work the foundation of the prepare position. Working the foundation of the pose is enough to build the strength required for a full inversion. Do not jump or kick the legs up. Work the steady strength of the foundational pose.

Try the Tripod "egg" position and walk the shinbones up along the shelf of the upper arms (see fig. 8.167). Do not use the wall for balance, but if necessary, use it for safety to prevent a hard crash. Do not place both feet against the wall or the torso will deviate from the center line. Stay for five breaths, then explore lifting the "egg" off the shelf of the upper arms by shifting the hips up and forward (see fig. 8.168). Press into the arms and firm the shoulder girdle, feel the center line, and activate the muscles of the pelvic floor to lift. Do not kick, jump, or push too hard. Stay for a few breaths, building up to five deep breaths, then return to the prepare position and come all the way down.

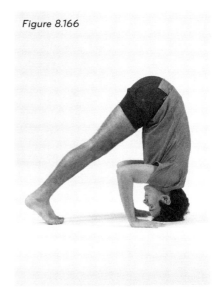

Figure 8.166

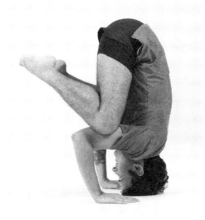

Figure 8.167

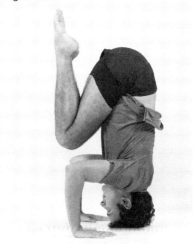

Figure 8.168

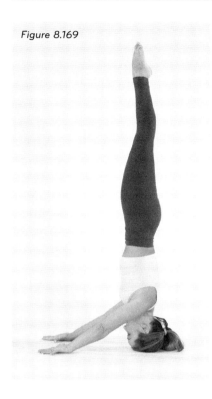

Figure 8.169

Mukta Hasta Sirsasana B
(Unsupported Headstand B)

CHAIR VARIATION

Start off seated in a chair. Stabilize the core of the body to feel the center line. Engage the pelvic floor, draw the muscles of the lower abdomen and the rib cage in toward the spine, and reach up and out through the top of the head. Draw the shoulder blades down the back and relax the neck. Inhale and let the arms drape down by the sides of the body. Keep the fingertips facing the ground, stabilize the shoulder girdle, straighten the elbows, and prepare the arm position for this headstand. Keep the arms forward in line with the shoulders. Either stay seated or stand up and work the alignment and shoulder strength of the pose without inverting (see fig. 8.170). Gaze toward the nose. Stay for five breaths, then return to seated. Between each of the headstands, flow through the vinyasa before proceeding to the next variation.

Try using a chair as support for the back and neck. Place a chair against a wall with the backrest of the chair facing the wall. Make sure the chair is secure and won't slide. Start on the hands and knees facing the chair and the wall. Engage the muscles of the pelvic floor, draw the muscles of the abdomen in toward the spine, draw the shoulder blades down the back, and stabilize the shoulder girdle and chest. Bend the knees and arms, and place the head on the floor just in front of the seat of the chair, almost in line with its front feet. Press the back against the seat of the chair. Inhale, straighten the legs up, and walk in to the tripod shape (see fig. 8.171). Switch the arms to the position of Mukta Hasta Sirsasana B. Straighten

Figure 8.170

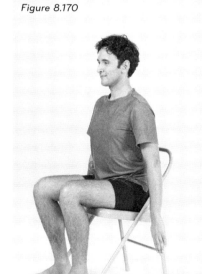

Figure 8.171

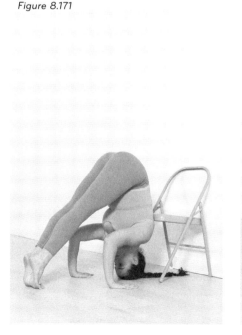

Figure 8.172

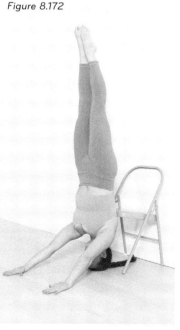

the arms in line with the shoulders, maintain the stability of the shoulder girdle and shoulder blades, and press the backs of the hands into the ground. If the body is not yet ready to invert fully, then stay here and work the foundation of the prepare position.

When the inversion feels accessible, inhale again and lift the legs to the center line of the body and find the balance (see fig. 8.172). Do not jump. If the balance is challenged, bend one knee and lightly touch the foot to the wall, but keep the other leg straight and in line with the torso. Do not place both feet against the wall or the torso will deviate from the center line. Stay for five breaths, then return to the prepare position and come all the way down.

FLOOR VARIATION

Start off on the hands and knees. Engage the muscles of the pelvic floor, draw the muscles of the abdomen in toward the spine, draw the shoulder blades down the back, and stabilize the shoulder girdle and chest. Bend the knees and arms, and place the head on the floor to form the tripod shape. Inhale, straighten the legs up, and walk in to the prepare position. Switch the arms to the position of Mukta Hasta Sirsasana B. Straighten the arms in line with the shoulders, maintain the stability of the shoulder girdle and shoulder blades, and press the backs of the hands into the ground (see fig. 8.173). If the body is not yet ready to invert fully, then stay here and work the foundation of the prepare position. Do not jump or kick the legs up. Work the steady strength of the foundational pose. Try lifting one leg to test strength and balance. Do not use the wall for balance, but if necessary, use it for safety to prevent a hard crash. If the balance is challenged, bend one knee and lightly touch the foot to the wall, but do not place both feet against the wall or the torso will deviate from the center line. Stay for five breaths, then return to the prepare position and come all the way down.

Figure 8.173

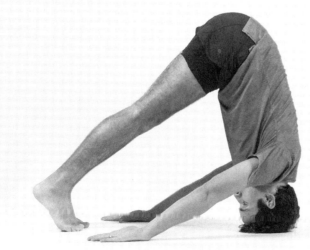

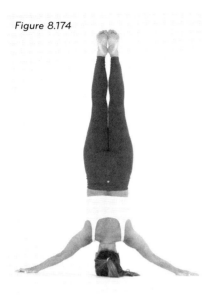

Figure 8.174

Mukta Hasta Sirsasana C
(Unsupported Headstand C)

CHAIR VARIATION

Start off seated in a chair. Stabilize the core of the body to feel the center line. Engage the pelvic floor, draw the muscles of the lower abdomen and the rib cage in toward the spine, and reach up and out through the top of the head. Draw the shoulder blades down the back and relax the neck. Inhale to lift the arms. Turn the palms up, extend the arms out to the sides to make a V shape, stabilize the shoulder girdle, straighten the elbows, and prepare the arm position for this headstand. Keep the arms in line with the shoulders and the plane of the torso. Either stay seated or stand up and work the alignment and shoulder strength of the pose without inverting (see fig. 8.175). Gaze toward the nose. Stay for five breaths, then return to seated. Between each of the headstands, flow through the vinyasa before proceeding to the next variation.

Try using a chair as support for the back and neck. Place a chair against a wall with the backrest of the chair facing the wall. Make sure the chair is secure and won't slide. Start on the hands and knees facing the chair and the wall. Engage the muscles of the pelvic floor, draw the muscles of the abdomen in toward the spine, draw the shoulder blades down the back, and stabilize the shoulder girdle and chest. Bend the knees and arms, and

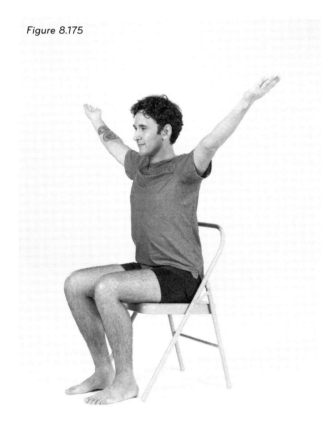

Figure 8.175

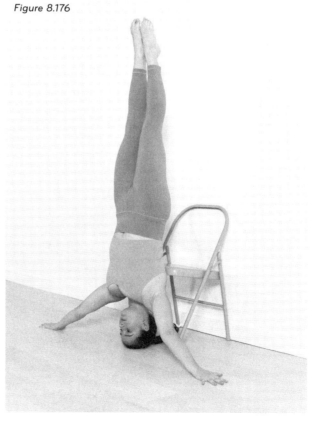

Figure 8.176

place the head on the floor just in front of the seat of the chair, almost in line with its front feet. Press the back against the seat of the chair. Inhale, straighten the legs up, and walk in to the tripod shape. Switch the arms to the position of Mukta Hasta Sirsasana C. Straighten the arms in line with the torso in a V shape, maintain the stability of the shoulder girdle and shoulder blades, and press the hands into the ground. If the body is not yet ready to invert fully, then stay here and work the foundation of the prepare position. When the inversion feels accessible, inhale again and lift the legs to the center line of the body and find the balance (see fig. 8.176). Do not jump. If the balance is challenged, bend one knee and lightly touch the foot to the wall, but keep the other leg straight and in line with the torso. Do not place both feet against the wall or the torso will deviate from the center line. Stay for five breaths, then return to the prepare position and come all the way down.

Figure 8.177

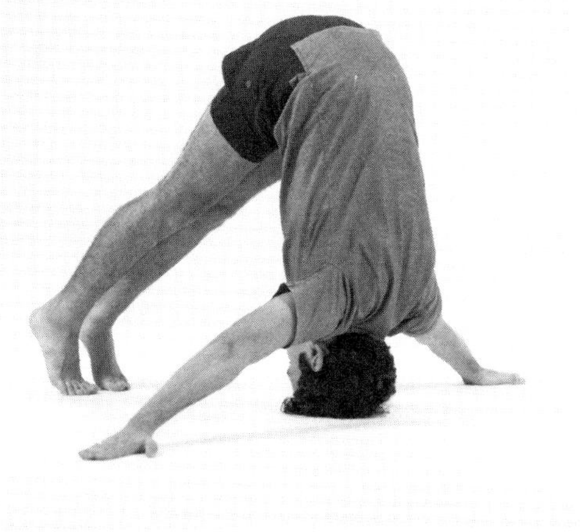

FLOOR VARIATION

Start off on the hands and knees. Engage the muscles of the pelvic floor, draw the muscles of the abdomen in toward the spine, draw the shoulder blades down the back, and stabilize the shoulder girdle and chest. Bend the knees and arms, and place the head on the floor to form the tripod shape. Inhale, straighten the legs up, and walk in to the prepare position. Switch the arms to the position of Mukta Hasta Sirsasana C. Straighten the arms in line with the torso out to the side, maintain the stability of the shoulder girdle and shoulder blades, and press the backs of the palms into the ground (see fig. 8.177). If the body is not yet ready to invert fully, then stay here and work the foundation of the prepare position. Do not jump or kick the legs up. Work the steady strength of the foundational pose. Try lifting one leg up to test strength and balance. Do not use the wall for balance, but if necessary, use it for safety to prevent a hard crash. If the balance is challenged, bend one knee and lightly touch the foot to the wall, but keep the other leg straight and in line with the torso. Do not place both feet against the wall or the torso will deviate from the center line. Stay for five breaths, then return to the prepare position and come all the way down.

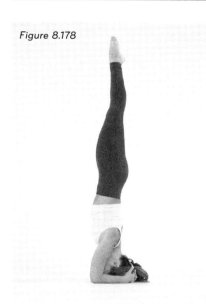

Figure 8.178

Baddha Hasta Sirsasana A (Bound Hands Headstand A)

These four headstands are considered the "supported headstands" and offer more support for the neck. However, do not be fooled into thinking these are easy; there is even more demand in terms of dynamic flexibility and strength. The body is challenged to stretch and stabilize simultaneously. Taken together, the unsupported and supported headstands—often referred to as "the seven headstands"—work to stabilize and harmonize the nervous system as well as run energy up the central channel. Approach whichever variation of these asanas is appropriate with respect and humility.

CHAIR VARIATION

Start off seated in a chair. Stabilize the core of the body to feel the center line. Engage the pelvic floor, draw the muscles of the lower abdomen and the rib cage in toward the spine, and reach up and out through the top of the head. Draw the shoulder blades down the back and relax the neck. Inhale to lift the arms. Bend the elbows to ninety degrees or slightly more. Wrap the hands around the back of the head and interlace the fingers to prepare the arm position for this headstand. Keep the elbows in line with the shoulders and do not allow them to splay out. Either stay seated or stand up and work the alignment and shoulder strength of the pose without inverting (see fig. 8.179). Gaze toward the nose. Stay for five breaths, then return to seated. Between each of the headstands, flow through the vinyasa before proceeding to the next variation.

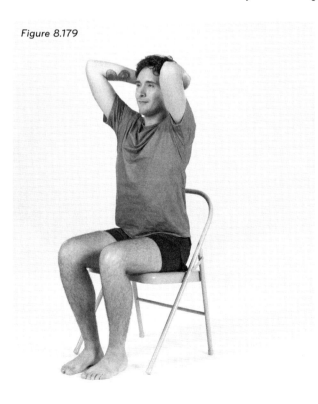

Figure 8.179

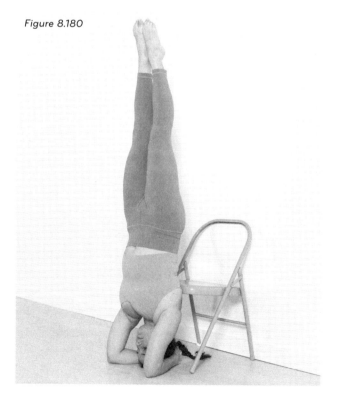

Figure 8.180

Try using a chair as support for the back and neck. Place a chair against a wall with the backrest of the chair facing the wall. Make sure the chair is secure and won't slide. Start on the hands and knees facing the chair and the wall. Engage the muscles of the pelvic floor, draw the muscles of the abdomen in toward the spine, draw the shoulder blades down the back, and stabilize the shoulder girdle and chest. Bend the knees and arms, and place the head on the floor just in front of the seat of the chair, almost in line with its front feet. Bend the elbows to ninety degrees or slightly more. Set the elbows down shoulder-width apart and interlace the fingers to prepare the arm position for this headstand by making a tripod base between the elbows and the palms. Note that this tripod is different than the tripod felt in the Mukta Hasta Sirsasana variations. Keep the elbows in line with the shoulders and do not allow them to splay out. Place the head down in the space between the hands to form a tripod between the elbows and the crown of the head. Press the back against the seat of the chair. Inhale, straighten the legs up, and walk the legs in as close to the head as possible. If the body is not yet ready to invert fully, then stay here and work the foundation of the prepare position. When the inversion feels accessible, inhale again and lift the legs to the center line of the body and find the balance (see fig. 8.180). Do not jump. If the balance is challenged, bend one knee and lightly touch the foot to the wall, but keep the other leg straight and in line with the torso. Do not place both feet against the wall or the torso will deviate from the center line. Stay for five breaths, then return to the prepare position and come all the way down.

FLOOR VARIATION

Start off on the hands and knees. Engage the muscles of the pelvic floor, draw the muscles of the abdomen in toward the spine, draw the shoulder blades down the back, and stabilize the shoulder girdle and chest. Place the head on the floor. Bend the elbows to ninety degrees or slightly more. Wrap the hands around the back of the head and interlace the fingers to prepare the arm position for this headstand. Keep the elbows in line with the shoulders and do not allow them to splay out. Inhale, straighten the legs up, and walk in as close to the head as possible (see fig. 8.181). If the body is not yet ready to invert fully, then stay here and work the foundation of the prepare position. Do not jump or kick the legs up. Work the steady strength of the foundational pose. Try lifting one leg to test strength and balance. Do not use the wall for balance, but if necessary, use it for safety to prevent a hard crash. If the balance is challenged, bend one knee and lightly touch the foot to the wall, but keep the other leg straight and in line with the torso. Do not place both feet against the wall or the torso will deviate from the center line. Stay for five breaths, then return to the prepare position and come all the way down.

Try Ardha Pincha Mayurasana and Makara Adho Mukha Svanasana as alternatives to build strength if the neck is not yet prepared for weight bearing.

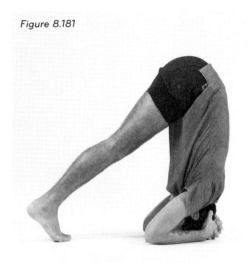

Figure 8.181

Figure 8.182

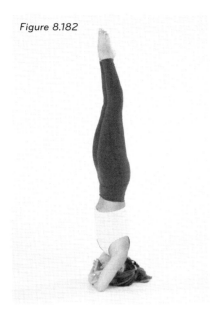

Baddha Hasta Sirsasana B
(Bound Hands Headstand B)

CHAIR VARIATION

Start off seated in a chair. Stabilize the core of the body to feel the center line. Engage the pelvic floor, draw the muscles of the lower abdomen and the rib cage in toward the spine, and reach up and out through the top of the head. Draw the shoulder blades down the back and relax the neck. Inhale to lift the arms. Bend the elbows to ninety degrees or slightly more. Wrap the hands around the opposite elbows, clasping the left bicep with the right hand and threading the left arm up and over the right to glide the left fingers around the right elbow nook. Keep the elbows in line with the shoulders and do not allow them to splay out. Either stay seated or stand up and work the alignment and shoulder strength of the pose without inverting (see fig. 8.183). Gaze toward the nose. Stay for five breaths, then return to seated. Between each of the headstands, flow through the vinyasa before proceeding to the next variation.

Try using a chair as support for the back and neck. Place a chair against a wall with the backrest of the chair facing the wall. Make sure the chair is secure and won't slide. Start on the hands and knees facing the chair and the wall. Engage the muscles of the pelvic floor, draw the muscles of the abdomen in toward the spine, draw the shoulder blades down the back, and stabilize the shoulder girdle and chest. Bend the knees and arms, and place the head on the floor just in front of the seat of the chair, almost in line

Figure 8.183

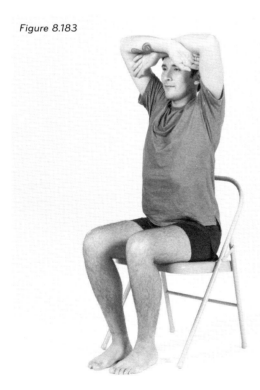

Figure 8.184

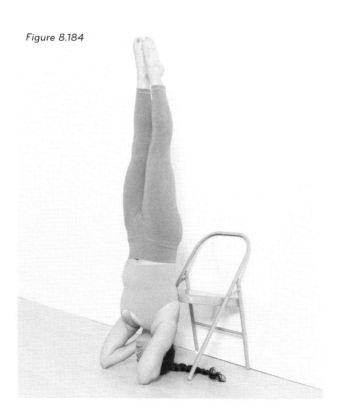

with its front feet. Bend the elbows to ninety degrees or slightly more. Wrap the hands around the opposite elbows, clasping the left bicep with the right hand and threading the left arm up and over the right to glide the left fingers around the right elbow nook. Keep the elbows in line with the shoulders and do not allow them to splay out. Place the head down in the same position on the floor as it was for the previous headstand but without the support of the hands around the head. The three points of contact with the ground create a tripod between the elbows and the crown of the head. Press the back against the seat of the chair. Inhale, straighten the legs up, and walk in as close to the head as possible. If the body is not yet ready to invert fully, then stay here and work the foundation of the prepare position. When the inversion feels accessible, inhale again and lift the legs to the center line of the body and find the balance (see fig. 8.184). Do not jump. If the balance is challenged, bend one knee and lightly touch the foot to the wall, but keep the other leg straight and in line with the torso. Do not place both feet against the wall or the torso will deviate from the center line. Stay for five breaths, then return to the prepare position and come all the way down.

Figure 8.185

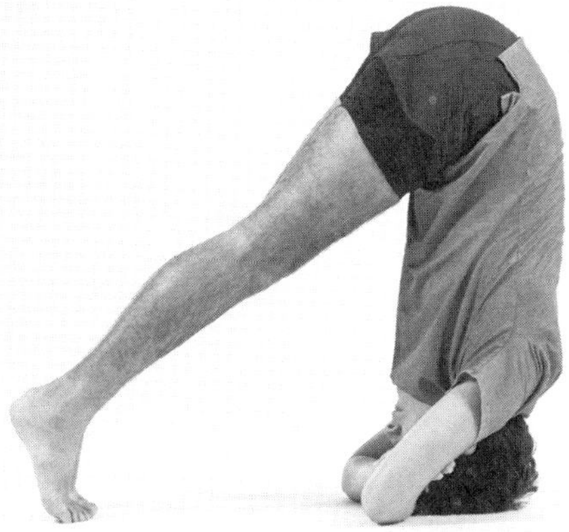

FLOOR VARIATION

Start off on the hands and knees. Engage the muscles of the pelvic floor, draw the muscles of the abdomen in toward the spine, draw the shoulder blades down the back, and stabilize the shoulder girdle and chest. Bend the elbows to ninety degrees or slightly more. Wrap the hands around the opposite elbows, clasping the left bicep with the right hand and threading the left arm up and over the right to glide the left fingers around the right elbow nook. Keep the elbows in line with the shoulders and do not allow them to splay out. Place the head down in the same position as it was for the previous headstand, creating the tripod base that all the bound-hand headstands have between the elbows and the crown of the head. Inhale, straighten the legs up, and walk in as close to the head as possible (see fig. 8.185). If the body is not yet ready to invert fully, then stay here and work the foundation of the prepare position. Do not jump or kick the legs up. Work the steady strength of the foundational pose. Try lifting one leg to test strength and balance. Do not use the wall for balance, but if necessary, use it for safety to prevent a hard crash. If the balance is challenged, bend one knee and lightly touch the foot to the wall, but keep the other leg straight and in line with the torso. Do not place both feet against the wall or the torso will deviate from the center line. Stay for five breaths, then return to the prepare position and come all the way down.

Try Ardha Pincha Mayurasana and Makara Adho Mukha Svanasana as alternatives to build strength if the neck is not yet prepared for weight bearing.

Figure 8.186

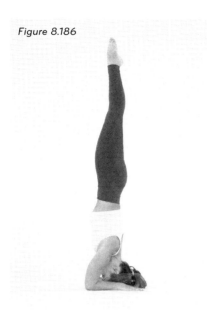

Baddha Hasta Sirsasana C
(Bound Hands Headstand C)

CHAIR VARIATION

Start off seated in a chair. Stabilize the core of the body to feel the center line. Engage the pelvic floor, draw the muscles of the lower abdomen and the rib cage in toward the spine, and reach up and out through the top of the head. Draw the shoulder blades down the back and relax the neck. Inhale to lift the arms. Bend the elbows to ninety degrees or slightly more. Align the hands either with the elbows or slightly in from the elbows. Do not grab the head. Keep the elbows in line with the shoulders and do not allow them to splay out. Either stay seated or stand up and work the alignment and shoulder strength of the pose without inverting (see fig. 8.187). Gaze toward the nose. Stay for five breaths, then return to seated. Between each of the headstands, flow through the vinyasa before proceeding to the next variation.

Try using a chair as support for the back and neck. Place a chair against a wall with the backrest of the chair facing the wall. Make sure the chair is secure and won't slide. Start on the hands and knees facing the chair and the wall. Engage the muscles of the pelvic floor, draw the muscles of the abdomen in toward the spine, draw the shoulder blades down the back, and stabilize the shoulder girdle and chest. Bend the knees and arms, and place the head on the floor just in front of the seat of the chair, almost in line with its front feet. Bend the elbows to ninety degrees or slightly more. Align the

Figure 8.187

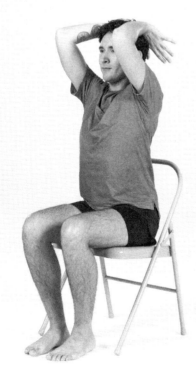

Figure 8.188

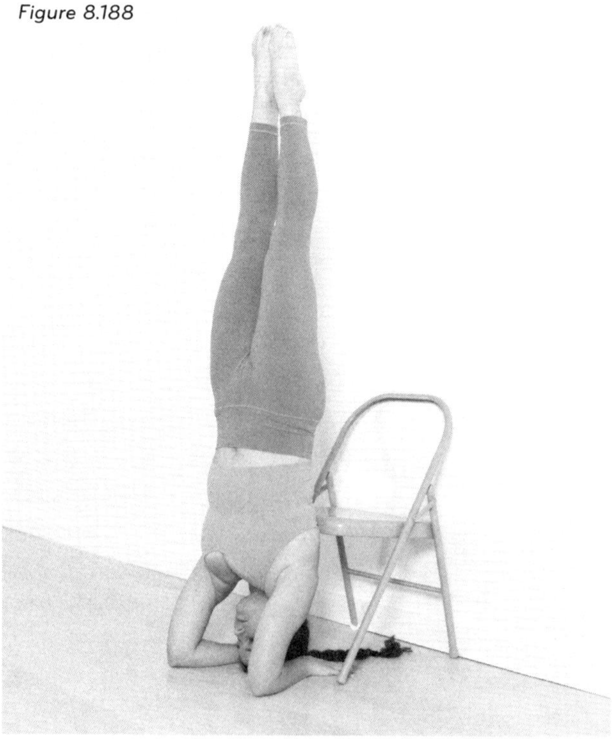

hands either with the elbows or slightly in from the elbows. Place the hands flat on the floor, and place the crown of the head on the floor between the hands. Do not grab the head. Press the back against the seat of the chair. Inhale, straighten the legs up, and walk in as close to the head as possible. If the body is not yet ready to invert fully, then stay here and work the foundation of the prepare position. When the inversion feels accessible, inhale again and lift the legs to the center line of the body and find the balance (see fig. 8.188). Do not jump. If the balance is challenged, bend one knee and lightly touch the foot to the wall, but keep the other leg straight and in line with the torso. Do not place both feet against the wall or the torso will deviate from the center line. Stay for five breaths, then return to the prepare position and come all the way down.

Figure 8.189

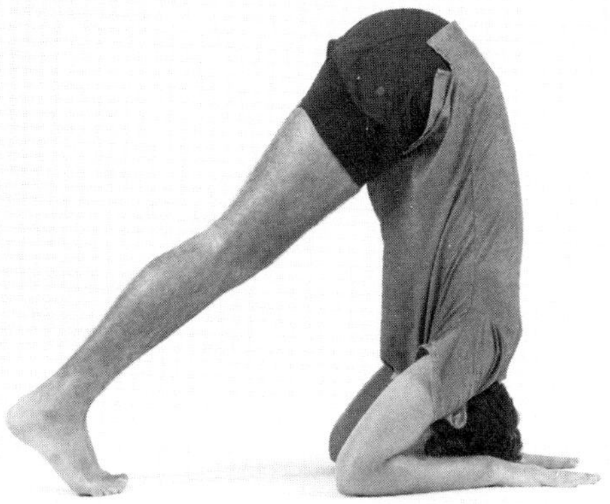

FLOOR VARIATION

Start off on the hands and knees. Engage the muscles of the pelvic floor, draw the muscles of the abdomen in toward the spine, draw the shoulder blades down the back, and stabilize the shoulder girdle and chest. Bend the elbows to ninety degrees or slightly more. Align the hands either with the elbows or slightly in from the elbows. Place the hands flat on the floor, and place the crown of the head on the floor between the hands. Do not grab the head. Inhale, straighten the legs up, and walk in as close to the head as possible (see fig. 8.189). If the body is not yet ready to invert fully, then stay here and work the foundation of the prepare position. Do not jump or kick the legs up. Work the steady strength of the foundational pose. Try lifting one leg to test strength and balance. Do not use the wall for balance, but if necessary, use it for safety to prevent a hard crash. If the balance is challenged, bend one knee and lightly touch the foot to the wall, but keep the other leg straight and in line with the torso. Do not place both feet against the wall or the torso will deviate from the center line. Stay for five breaths, then return to the prepare position and come all the way down.

Try Ardha Pincha Mayurasana and Makara Adho Mukha Svanasana as alternatives to build strength if the neck is not yet prepared for weight bearing.

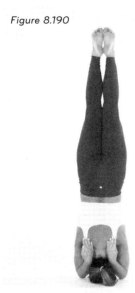

Figure 8.190

Baddha Hasta Sirsasana D
(Bound Hands Headstand D)

CHAIR VARIATION

Start off seated in a chair. Stabilize the core of the body to feel the center line. Engage the pelvic floor, draw the muscles of the lower abdomen and the rib cage in toward the spine, and reach up and out through the top of the head. Draw the shoulder blades down the back and relax the neck. Inhale to lift the arms. Bend the elbows to almost fully close the elbow joints. Slide the hands up along the trapezius muscles, but do not hold on to them. Close the fingers and let the hands rest along the upper inner line of the back. Keep the elbows in line with or slightly in from the shoulders, and do not allow them to splay out. Either stay seated or stand up and work the alignment and shoulder strength of the pose without inverting (see fig. 8.191). Gaze toward the nose. Stay for five breaths, then return to seated. Between each of the headstands, flow through the vinyasa before proceeding to the next variation.

Try using a chair as support for the back and neck. Place a chair against a wall with the backrest of the chair facing the wall. Make sure the chair is secure and won't slide. Start on the hands and knees facing the chair and the wall. Engage the muscles of the pelvic floor, draw the muscles of the abdomen in toward the spine, draw the shoulder blades down the back, and stabilize the shoulder girdle and chest. Bend the knees and arms, and place the head on the floor just in front of the seat of the chair, almost in

Figure 8.191

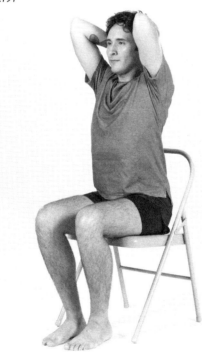

Figure 8.192

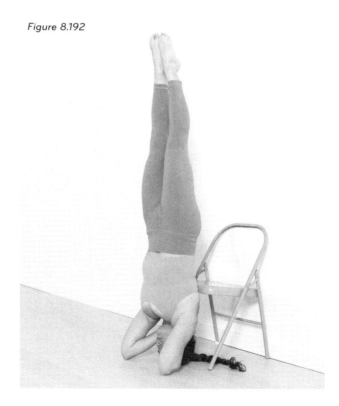

line with its front feet. Bend the elbows to almost fully close the elbow joints. Slide the hands up along the trapezius muscles, but do not hold on to them. Close the fingers and let the hands rest along the upper inner line of the back. Align the elbows with the shoulders and actively press down into the ground through the elbows. Place the head on the floor to form a tripod between the elbows and the crown of the head. Keep the elbows in line with or slightly in from the shoulders, and do not allow them to splay out. Press the back against the seat of the chair. Inhale, straighten the legs up, and walk in as close to the head as possible. If the body is not yet ready to invert fully, then stay here and work the foundation of the prepare position. When the inversion feels accessible, inhale again and lift the legs to the center line of the body and find the balance (see fig. 8.192). Do not jump. If the balance is challenged, bend one knee and lightly touch the foot to the wall, but keep the other leg straight and in line with the torso. Do not place both feet against the wall or the torso will deviate from the center line. Stay for five breaths, then return to the prepare position and come all the way down.

Figure 8.193

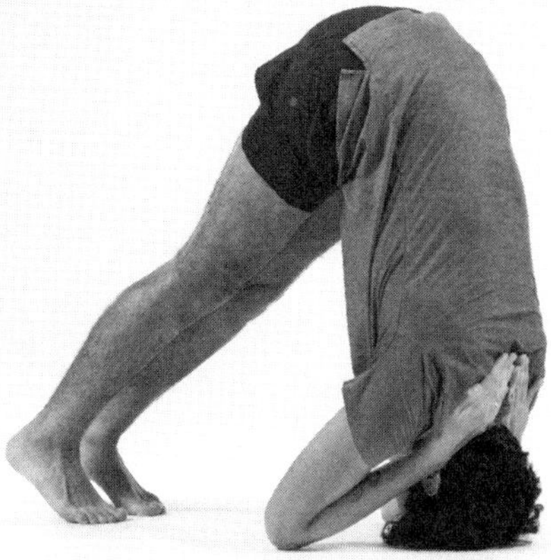

FLOOR VARIATION

Start off on the hands and knees. Engage the muscles of the pelvic floor, draw the muscles of the abdomen in toward the spine, draw the shoulder blades down the back, and stabilize the shoulder girdle and chest. Bend the elbows to almost fully close the elbow joints. Slide the hands up along the trapezius muscles, but do not hold on to them. Close the fingers and let the hands rest along the upper inner line of the back. Align the elbows with the shoulders and actively press down into the ground through the elbows. Place the head on the floor to form a tripod between the elbows and the crown of the head. Keep the elbows in line with or slightly in from the shoulders, and do not allow them to splay out. Inhale, straighten the legs up, and walk in as close to the head as possible (see fig. 8.193). If the body is not yet ready to invert fully, then stay here and work the foundation of the prepare position. Do not jump or kick the legs up. Work the steady strength of the foundational pose. Try lifting one leg to test strength and balance. Do not use the wall for balance, but if necessary, use it for safety to prevent a hard crash. If the balance is challenged, bend one knee and lightly touch the foot to the wall, but keep the other leg straight and in line with the torso. Do not place both feet against the wall or the torso will deviate from the center line. Stay for five breaths, then return to the prepare position and come all the way down.

Try Ardha Pincha Mayurasana and Makara Adho Mukha Svanasana as alternatives to build strength if the neck is not yet prepared for weight bearing.

Backbends &
Closing Poses

VERY YOGA PRACTICE leaves a residue in the body and mind. The subtle elements of matter and spirit synergize with each breath and each asana. While Ashtanga Yoga comprises six series of poses, all students of this discipline always include Sun Salutations, Standing Poses, and Closing Poses in their daily practice. Backbends are usually also part of every practice; however, K. Pattabhi Jois always said that a complete practice can include only the Sun Salutations, Standing Poses, and the last three seated asanas of the Closing Poses. In this way, the practice is always adaptable and accommodating for days when you may not have lots of time, when the body feels tired or injured, or whenever it just feels better to do a shorter practice. Rather than set the goal of practice to be an unattainable high where you do either ninety minutes to two hours of sweaty, intense asanas or nothing at all, it's better to do what you can with the time you have. Just as the poses can be adapted, so can the length of the practice. But no matter how long or short the practice may be on any given day, it is important to end each practice with a high level of integrity and integrate the spiritual lessons of each practice.

BACKBENDS

Backbending is its own mini-practice within the practice, and it holds a whole series of trials and tribulations for all students regardless of their level of natural flexibility. More than a contortive performance, backbending in yoga is not just about pushing the spine to increasingly extreme degrees. Instead, the effort of spinal extension stimulates subtle energy centers that sit along the central axis of the body. The energy of backbending starts at the soles of the feet; moves through the tailbone or sacrum, the navel, the sternum, the arms, the throat, and the eyebrows; and ends at the top of the head. Involving every muscle of the body in a carefully orchestrated series of muscular recruitments and releases, backbending brings up emotional, mental, and physical obstacles. Cultivating an attitude of nonattachment, equanimity, compassion, and wisdom is crucial to traversing the tumultuous ocean of backbending. Every student who works backbending with respect for the body will experience the benefits of increased energy flow, heightened sensory perception, a more balanced nervous system, improved cardiovascular function, and more. Focus on the subtlety of the inner work and release the need to achieve any particular shape in any particular time. The opening of the spine and the accompanying subtle energy centers cannot be rushed. The benefits of backbending are available for every student who applies the technique with diligence and determination.

Urdhva Dhanurasana (Lifted Bow Pose)

Figure 9.1

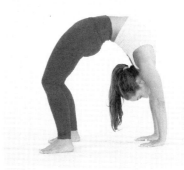

CHAIR VARIATION

Start off seated in a chair facing the backrest. Slide the feet through the empty space between the backrest and the seat. Align the feet hip-width or slightly wider apart. Clasp the sides of the backrest. Inhale and engage the muscles of the pelvic floor, draw the muscles of the abdomen in toward the spine, lift the ribs away from the hips, and stabilize the legs. Exhale and gently bend backward. While the middle and lower back are supported by the seat of the chair, allow the upper back to cascade over the end of the seat and drop the neck back (see fig. 9.2). If the seat feels too hard, place a blanket or cushion on it to add more padding. If the body feels comfortable and the breath is relaxed and flowing, extend the arms over the head and place the palms on the floor. Externally rotate the shoulders and align

Figure 9.2

Figure 9.3

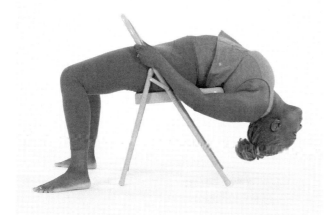

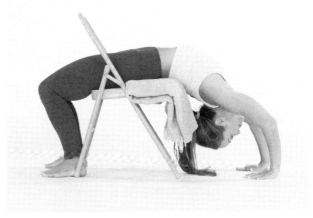

the elbows with the shoulders to avoid splaying the arms out to the sides. Gently shift the gaze toward the space between the hands on the floor (see fig. 9.3). Stay for five breaths, then return to seated. Repeat three times.

FLOOR VARIATIONS

Urdhva Dhanurasana is often referred to as Bridge Pose in many other styles of yoga. Accordingly, working on increasing spinal extension and front-body range of motion from various forms of this pose is a great way to adapt backbending to suit the practice. Find the option that best supports the body's ability to do the inner work of yoga. It may be advisable to work through all the options suggested here to progressively deepen the body's ability to bend backward. Practice slowly without attachment to a particular result.

Start off lying down. Bend the knees and align the feet hip-width apart. Inhale and engage the muscles of the pelvic floor, draw the muscles of the abdomen in toward the spine, lift the ribs away from the hips, and engage the quadriceps. Place a block under the sacrum, extend the arms out, and relax the glutes (see fig. 9.4). Check in with how the body feels. There should be no compression or crunching sensations in the spine or any of the vertebrae. If the body feels good, consider lifting off the block. Roll the shoulders under the back and internally rotate the shoulder joints. Reach along the length of the body to clasp the ankles (see fig. 9.5). Stay for five breaths, then return to lying down. Repeat three times.

Figure 9.4

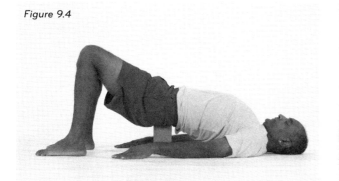

Figure 9.5

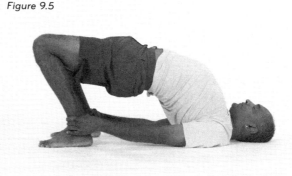

Try a more intense version of this pose with a strap to support shoulder alignment. Lie down, wrap a strap around the elbows, and adjust the strap to hold the arms shoulder-width apart. Bend the knees and align the feet hip-width apart. Engage the muscles of the pelvic floor, draw the muscles of the abdomen in toward the spine, lift the ribs away from the hips, and engage the quadriceps. Lift the arms above the head, bend the elbows, and place the palms on the floor with the fingers pointing toward the feet. Inhale and lift the hips, then the torso, to roll onto the top of the head (see fig. 9.6). Stay here for a few breaths. If this is enough, then come down, but if the body feels good, try straightening the arms. Inhale again and

Figure 9.6

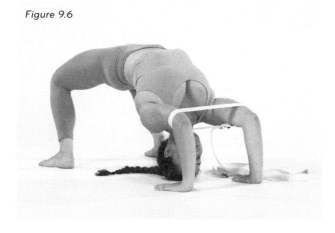

Figure 9.8

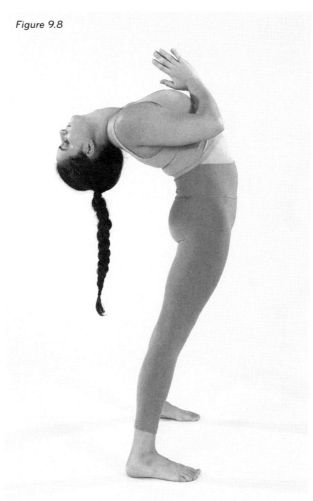

Figure 9.7

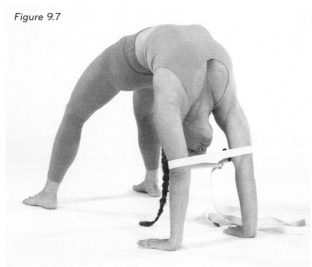

increase the activation of the muscles along the back of the body and the legs. Draw the elbows in toward each other and gaze between the hands (see fig. 9.7). Maximize the space between the ribs and the hips. Stay for five breaths, then repeat three times. If the neck feels safe and supported, come down only onto the top of the head between repetitions; otherwise, come all the way down.

Standing up and dropping back into Urdhva Dhanurasana can be extremely challenging. However, working a spinal extension from standing can be both accessible and deeply beneficial. Start off standing with the feet hip-width or slightly wider apart and keeping them parallel. Place the hands in prayer position at the center of the chest. Inhale and engage the muscles of the pelvic floor, draw the muscles of the abdomen in toward the spine, lift the ribs away from the hips, and engage the quadriceps. Exhale and engage the back muscles to slowly arch backward. Once the shoulders shift forward and a nice arch occurs, gently drop the head back (see fig. 9.8). Look for the floor. Stay for five breaths, then return to standing. Repeat three times.

Figure 9.9

Figure 9.10

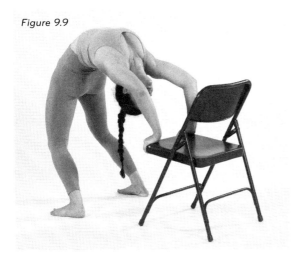

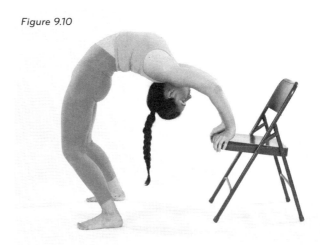

Try another version with a chair, a sofa, or the wall. Stand in front of the chair, facing away from it. Repeat all the instructions already outlined for the standing backbend. Once the chair (or other supportive object) is visible, go on to the next step. If the chair is not within the line of vision, do not proceed. Make sure the chair is secure on the floor. Continuing from the standing backbend, inhale again and extend the arms over the head, following the line of the backbend. Do not lift the arms up toward the ceiling but toward the chair. Maintain the external rotation of the shoulders. Exhale and gently bend the knees to drop the hands back to the seat of the chair (see figs. 9.9 and 9.10). Stay for a breath to settle. If the legs feel weak, then bend the knees and sit down. If the legs feel strong, engage the quadriceps even more to root down through the feet. Inhale and shift the hips forward to return to standing. Repeat three times.

CLOSING POSES

To soak in the deep benefits of the practice, finish with at least a few of the following integrative asanas each time you step on the mat. Longer holds in inverted poses help the nervous system settle. Emphasize deep, resonant breathing even more throughout this part of the practice than anywhere else. Extend the breath and reach toward a ten-second inhalation and exhalation. Yoga works in more ways than are apparent on the surface. The analytical mind is not always aware of the subtle changes transpiring in the deeper regions of the mind. The Closing Poses help bridge the gap between the conscious and the subconscious mind. More than just a cool-down, this series is a spiritual practice that stimulates mystical centers in the brain and the subtle body. Do not skip over or rush through this portion of the practice. Let it take the time it takes so when you get to the final relaxation at the end, your entire being will be transported to a blissful state beyond words. Allow the hard edges to soften. Explore the outer limits of consciousness. Release more and more into the Infinite.

Salamba Sarvangasana (Shoulderstand)

Figure 9.11

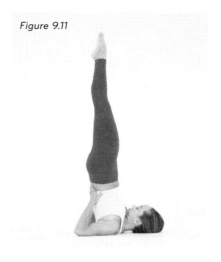

CHAIR VARIATION

While it is not advisable to invert while seated in a chair, it is possible to lie on a sofa or bed and elevate the legs. If lying on the floor is accessible, try using the chair for stability and alignment. Lie down in front of the chair. Bend the knees into the chest, and scoot the hips toward the front legs of the chair. Hold on to the front legs of the chair near the feet. Once the hands have a firm grip, inhale and straighten and lift the legs, allowing the seat of the chair to support the backs of the legs (see fig. 9.12). Engage the muscles of the pelvic floor; draw the muscles of the lower abdomen in toward the spine; activate the quadriceps; and relax the head, neck, and torso. Gaze toward the nose or the toes. Stay for ten to twenty-five breaths. Then either come down or proceed immediately to the next pose in the shoulderstand sequence.

FLOOR VARIATIONS

Start off lying on the floor. Bend the knees and place a block, blanket, or bolster under the sacrum. Engage the muscles of the pelvic floor; draw the muscles of the lower abdomen in toward the spine; activate the quadriceps; and relax the head, neck, and torso. Lift the legs to form a ninety-degree angle between the legs and the torso (see fig. 9.13). Place the hands on the floor by the sides of the body. Gaze toward the nose or the toes. Point or flex the feet, whichever feels more stabilizing. Stay for ten to twenty-five breaths. Then either come down or proceed immediately to the next pose in the shoulderstand sequence. To provide added support, this pose can also be done against the wall or a strap can be tied around the legs. Explore the options that work best for the body.

Figure 9.12

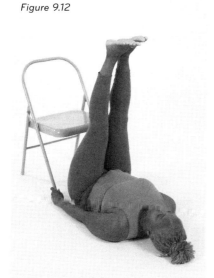

Figure 9.13

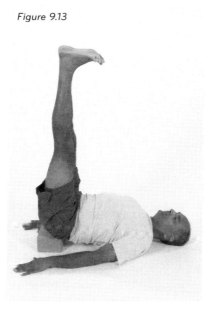

Figure 9.14

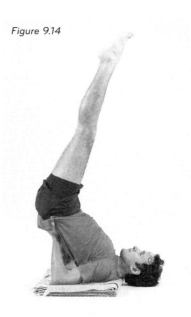

Try making a V shape with the support of blankets (see fig. 9.14). Settle the shoulders and upper body over two folded blankets. Roll the shoulder blades gently down the back and away from each other, draw the elbows in to align with the shoulders, allow the neck to be free, and let the head float toward the floor beyond the blankets. Inhale and lift the body with the strength of the pelvic floor muscles. Draw the muscles of the abdomen in toward the spine, engage the quadriceps, and bring the legs together. Rest the sacrum and lower back in the palms. Breathe deeply, and gaze toward either the nose or the feet.

Figure 9.15

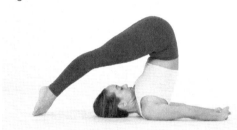

Halasana (Plow Pose)

CHAIR VARIATION

This variation is not advisable for individuals who cannot get up from and down to the floor comfortably. Start off lying down in front of a chair. Place a folded blanket or large towel under the shoulders. Engage the muscles of the pelvic floor, and draw the muscles of the lower abdomen in toward the spine. Roll the shoulders under the body and internally rotate the shoulders to use the trapezius muscles to give space to the head and neck. Hold on to a strap with both hands to stabilize the shoulders and gently guide the hands toward the floor, behind the back. Keep the hands as close to shoulder-width apart as possible or slightly narrower than shoulder-width apart (it is not necessary to try to force the hands to touch the floor). Inhale and activate the quadriceps to lift the legs up and over the body; rest the feet on the seat of the chair. Lift the hips up in line with the shoulders or as close to the line of the shoulders as possible (see fig. 9.16). Stay for five to ten breaths, then either come down or proceed immediately with the rest of the shoulderstand sequence.

Figure 9.16

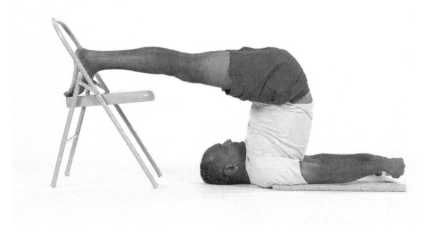

Figure 9.17

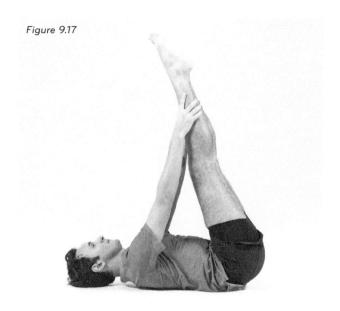

Figure 9.18

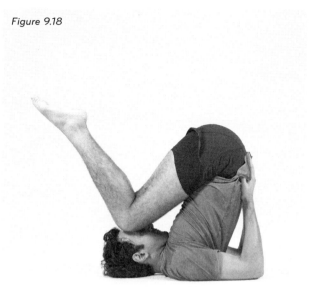

FLOOR VARIATION

Continuing from Salamba Sarvangasana, explore which option best supports the body. If the back is resting on the floor, reach the arms up toward the shinbones and gently lift the hips off the ground to facilitate a forward fold (see fig. 9.17). Stay for five to ten breaths. Gaze toward the nose or up toward the feet. If continuing from the V shape feels good, gently allow the feet to drop closer to the floor over the head throughout the five to ten breaths of the pose. Sometimes bending the knees and dropping the kneecaps toward the head is a good option if the hamstrings are too tight (see fig. 9.18).

Karnapidasana (Ear Pressure Pose)

While this asana may seem very intimidating, there are ways to approach and adapt it that can make the practice accessible. Try Ananda Balasana or Supta Baddha Konasana as alternatives.

Figure 9.19

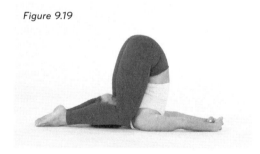

FLOOR VARIATION

Continuing directly from Halasana, engage the muscles of the pelvic floor and draw the muscles of the lower abdomen in toward the spine. Roll the shoulders under the body and internally rotate the shoulders to use the trapezius muscles to give space to the head and neck. Keep holding on to a strap with both hands to stabilize the shoulders and gently guide the hands toward the floor behind the back in the same manner as in Sarvangasana (again, it is not necessary to try to force the hands to touch the floor). Inhale and lift the legs up and over the body, bend the knees, and gently engage the inner thighs to place light pressure on the ears or in the direction of the ears. Sometimes it is beneficial to release the strap

Figure 9.20

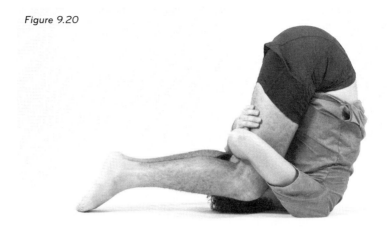

and place the hands around the backs of the knees to support the weight distribution of the body closer to the center line (see fig. 9.20). Place a blanket or large towel folded up under the shoulders if there is a lot of undue pressure on the neck, shoulders, or upper back. Stay for five to ten breaths, then either come down or proceed immediately with the rest of the shoulderstand sequence.

Figure 9.21

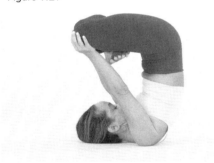

Figure 9.22

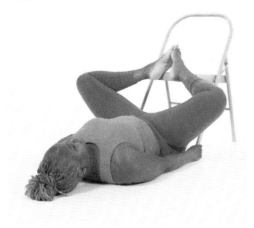

Urdhva Padmasana (Flying Lotus Pose)

CHAIR VARIATION

While it is not advisable to invert while seated in a chair, it is possible to lie on a sofa or bed and elevate the legs. If lying on the floor is accessible, try using the chair for stability and alignment. Lie down in front of the chair or continue directly from the shoulderstand sequence. Bend the knees into the chest, and scoot the hips toward the front legs of the chair. Hold on to the chair legs near the feet. Once the hands have a firm grip, inhale and lift the legs, allowing the seat of the chair to support the backs of the legs (see fig. 9.22). Draw the feet toward each other and externally rotate the hip joints. This may feel like an elevated variation of Supta Baddha Konasana. Engage the muscles of the pelvic floor; draw the muscles of the lower abdomen in toward the spine; activate the quadriceps; and relax the head, neck, and torso. Gaze toward the nose or toward the toes. Stay for five to ten breaths, then either come down or proceed immediately with the next pose in the shoulderstand sequence.

FLOOR VARIATION

Lie down on the back. Fold the legs into a lotus position or cross them at the shinbones. Engage the muscles of the pelvic floor; draw the muscles of the lower abdomen in toward the spine; and relax the head, neck, and torso. Bend the knees and lift the legs to form an approximately ninety-degree

Figure 9.23

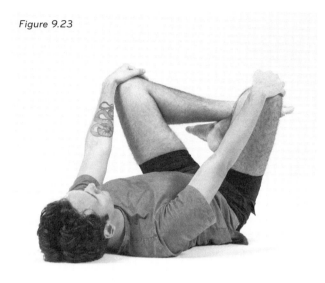

Figure 9.24

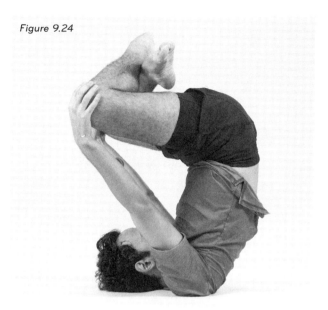

angle in the hip joints. Extend the arms toward the knees and press firmly down to replicate the sensation of lifting into Padmasana with the hands resting on the knees in Salamba Sarvangasana (see fig. 9.23). Gaze toward the nose or the toes. If balance feels good in Salamba Sarvangasana but Padmasana remains inaccessible, try balancing in a cross-legged position instead (see fig. 9.24) Stay for five to ten breaths, then either exit the pose or proceed immediately to the next pose in the shoulderstand sequence.

Pindasana (Embryo Pose)

Figure 9.25

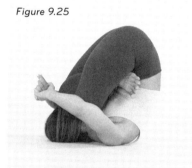

CHAIR VARIATION

While it is not advisable to invert while seated in a chair, it is possible to lie on a sofa or bed and elevate the legs. If lying on the floor is accessible, try using the chair for stability and alignment. Lie down in front of the chair or continue directly from the shoulderstand sequence. Bend the knees into the chest and scoot the hips toward the front legs of the chair. Hold on to the chair legs near the feet. Once the hands have a firm grip, inhale and lift the legs, allowing the seat of the chair to support the backs of the legs. Engage the muscles of the pelvic floor; draw the muscles of the lower abdomen in toward the spine; activate the quadriceps; and relax the head, neck, and torso. Gently lift the feet off the chair and fold the thighs in toward the torso. Wrap the hands around the shins; interlace the fingers or hold the shinbones (see fig. 9.26). Gaze toward the nose or the toes. Stay for five to ten breaths, then either come down or proceed immediately to the next pose in the shoulderstand sequence.

Figure 9.26

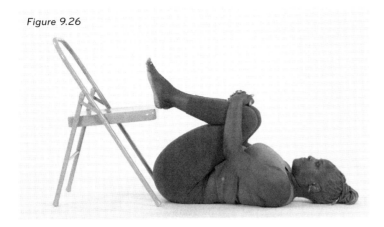

Figure 9.27

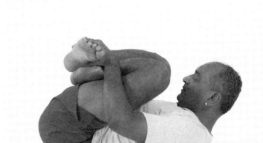

Figure 9.28

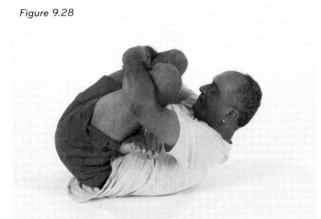

Figure 9.29

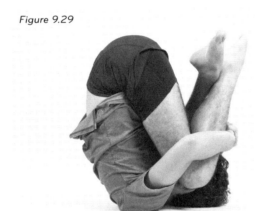

FLOOR VARIATION

Lie down on the back. Fold the legs into a lotus position or cross them at the shinbones. Engage the muscles of the pelvic floor; draw the muscles of the lower abdomen in toward the spine; and relax the head, neck, and torso. Bend the knees and lift the legs into the torso. Hug the legs firmly and lift the head to form a tight ball (see figs. 9.27 and 9.28). If the neck feels unsafe or unsupported while it's lifted, leave it resting on the floor or on a blanket or block. Gaze toward the nose or close the eyes. If the body feels comfortable in Salamba Sarvangasana but Padmasana is inaccessible, try folding the body into a tightly knit ball with the legs crossed while remaining inverted (see fig. 9.29). Stay for five to ten breaths, then either exit the pose or proceed immediately to the next pose in the shoulderstand sequence.

Matysasana (Fish Pose)

Figure 9.30

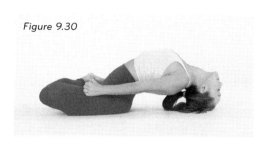

CHAIR VARIATION

While it is not advisable to invert while seated in a chair, it is possible to lie on a sofa or bed and elevate the legs. If lying on the floor is accessible, try using the chair for stability and alignment. Lie down in front of the chair or continue directly from the shoulderstand sequence. Bend the knees into the chest, and scoot the hips toward the front legs of the chair. Hold on to the chair legs near the feet. Once the hands have a firm grip, inhale and lift the legs, allowing the seat of the chair to support the backs of the legs. Engage the muscles of the pelvic floor; draw the muscles of the lower abdomen in toward the spine; activate the quadriceps; and relax the head, neck, and torso. Externally rotate the hip joints and point the soles of the feet toward each other. Bend the elbows, internally rotate the shoulders, and take the hands to the glutes just under the iliac crests (see figs. 9.31 and 9.32). Allow the head to be supported by the trapezius muscles, or place a bolster under the head for extra support. Gaze toward the nose or close the eyes. Stay for five to ten breaths, then either come down or proceed immediately to the next pose in the shoulderstand sequence.

Figure 9.31

Figure 9.32

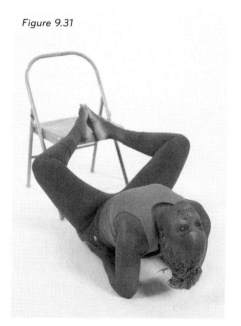

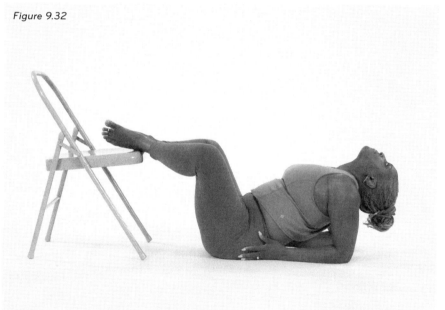

FLOOR VARIATION

Roll the spine gently down from whichever variation of Salamba Sarvangasana is appropriate. Once fully reclining, prepare to enter the pose. Working without the legs in the lotus position, cross the shinbones, engage the pelvic floor, and draw the muscles of the abdomen in toward the spine. Inhale and lift the rib cage. Use the elbows to prop the upper back and shoulders up, lift the upper spine off the floor, and arch the head back.

Figure 9.33

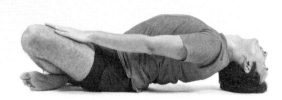

Figure 9.34

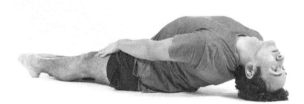

Figure 9.35

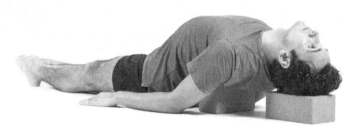

Once the head comfortably settles onto the floor, extend the arms and place the palms on the thighs (see fig. 9.33). Extending the legs is another option if the knees are sore (see fig. 9.34). If the neck and spine need support, try this variation with two blocks. Organize the blocks into a T shape so the blocks are perpendicular to each other. Place the head on the block that holds the long neck of the T shape and the upper back on the top edge (see fig. 9.35). Be sure the body feels fully supported. Gaze toward the nose. Stay for five to ten breaths and continue immediately into the next pose.

Figure 9.36

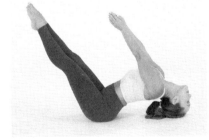

Uttana Padasana (Extended-Foot Pose)

CHAIR VARIATION

While it is not advisable to invert while seated in a chair, it is possible to lie on a sofa or bed and elevate the legs. If lying on the floor is accessible, try using the chair for stability and alignment. Lie down in front of the chair or continue directly from the shoulderstand sequence. Bend the knees into the chest, and scoot the hips toward the front legs of the chair. Hold on to the chair legs near the feet. Once the hands have a firm grip, inhale and lift the legs, allowing the seat of the chair to support the backs of the legs. Engage the muscles of the pelvic floor; draw the muscles of the lower abdomen in toward the spine; activate the quadriceps; and relax the head, neck, and torso. Internally rotate the hip joints and draw the legs toward each other. Bend the elbows, internally rotate the shoulders, and take the

Figure 9.37

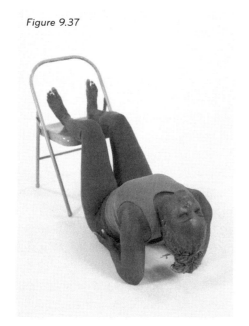

Figure 9.38

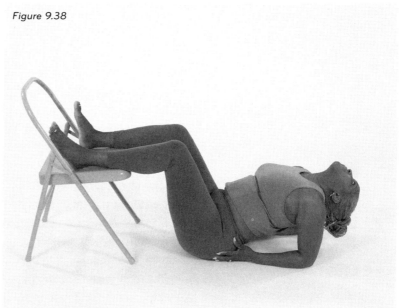

hands to the glutes just under the iliac crests (see figs. 9.37 and 9.38). Allow the head to be supported by the trapezius muscles, or place a bolster under the head for extra support. Gaze toward the nose or close the eyes. Stay for five to ten breaths, then come down and prepare for the next pose.

FLOOR VARIATION

If the head and neck feel comfortable in the arched position, continue directly into this pose. Extend the arms so the palms touch. Bend the knees, point the toes, and maintain the same head and neck position as in Matsyasana (see fig. 9.39). If the neck and upper back feel unsafe or require more support, flatten the back completely before proceeding. Once the head and back fully settle into the ground, extend the arms, touch the palms together, and gently bend the knees. If the lower back feels strong enough, lift the legs off the ground and straighten them (see fig. 9.40). Gaze toward the nose. Stay for five to ten breaths, then come down and prepare for the next pose.

Figure 9.39

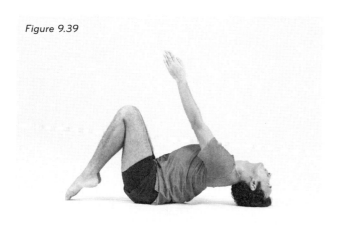

Figure 9.40

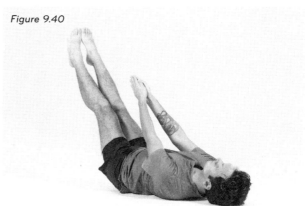

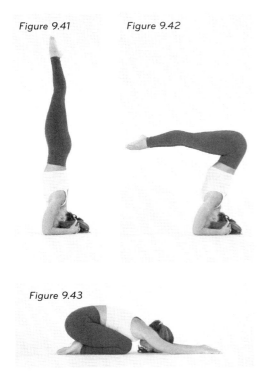

Figure 9.41   Figure 9.42

Figure 9.43

Sirsasana (Headstand)

CHAIR VARIATION

Start off seated in a chair. Stabilize the core of the body to feel the center line. Engage the pelvic floor, draw the muscles of the lower abdomen and the rib cage in toward the spine, and reach up and out through the top of the head. Draw the shoulder blades down the back and relax the neck. Inhale to lift the arms. Bend the elbows to almost fully close the elbow joints. Align the elbows with the shoulders and actively press down upward through the elbows to mimic the feeling of pressing into the floor. Keep the elbows in line with or slightly in from the shoulders, and do not allow them to splay out. Either stay seated or stand up and work the alignment and shoulder strength of the pose without inverting (see fig. 9.44). Gaze toward the nose. Stay for five breaths, then return to seated.

Try using a chair as support for the back and neck. Place a chair against a wall with the backrest of the chair facing the wall. Make sure the chair is secure and won't slide. Start on the hands and knees facing the chair and the wall. Engage the muscles of the pelvic floor, draw the muscles of the abdomen in toward the spine, draw the shoulder blades down the back, and stabilize the shoulder girdle and chest. Bend the knees and arms, and place the head on the floor just in front of the seat of the chair, almost in line with its front feet. Bend the elbows to almost fully close the elbow joints. Align the elbows with the shoulders and actively press down into

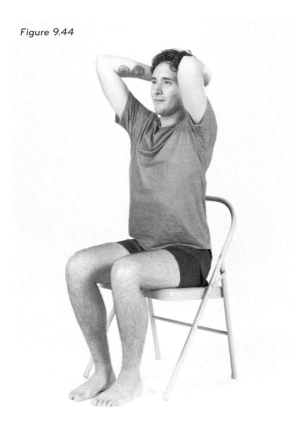

Figure 9.44

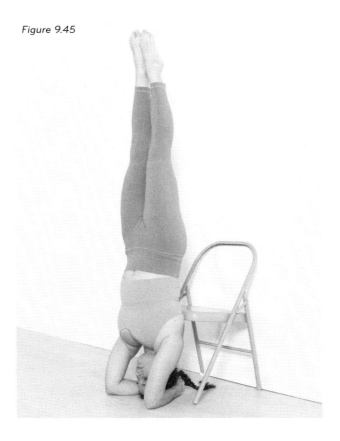

Figure 9.45

the ground through the elbows. Interlace the fingers and keep a small space to place the head between the open palms. Place the head on the floor to form a tripod between the elbows and the crown of the head. Keep the elbows in line with or slightly in from the shoulders, and do not allow them to splay out or lift up off the ground. Press the back against the seat of the chair. Inhale, straighten the legs up, and walk in as close to the head as possible. If the body is not yet ready to invert fully, then stay here and work the foundation of the prepare position. When the inversion feels accessible, inhale again and lift the legs to the center line of the body and find the balance (see fig. 9.45). Do not jump. If the balance is challenged, bend one knee and lightly touch the foot to the wall, but keep the other leg straight and in line with the torso. Do not place both feet against the wall or the torso will deviate from the center line. Stay for ten to twenty-five breaths, then return to the prepare position and come all the way down. Rest in Balasana for five breaths.

Adapt Balasana to the chair. Sit in the chair with the feet hip-width apart, fold the torso forward, and drape the arms down the sides of the legs.

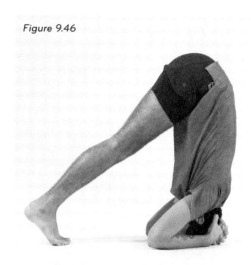

Figure 9.46

FLOOR VARIATION

Start off on the hands and knees. Engage the muscles of the pelvic floor, draw the muscles of the abdomen in toward the spine, draw the shoulder blades down the back, and stabilize the shoulder girdle and chest. Bend the knees and arms, interlace the fingers, and keep a small space to place the head between the open palms. Place the head on the floor in the space between the palms to form a tripod between the elbows and the crown of the head. Align the elbows with the shoulders and actively press down into the ground through the elbows. Keep the elbows in line with or slightly in from the shoulders, and do not allow them to splay out or lift up off the ground. Inhale, straighten the legs up, and walk in as close to the head as possible (see fig.9.46). If the body is not yet ready to invert fully, then stay here and work the foundation of the prepare position. Do not jump or kick the legs up. Work the steady strength of the foundational pose. Try lifting one leg to test strength and balance. Do not use the wall for balance, but if necessary, use it for safety to prevent a hard crash. If the balance is challenged, bend one knee and lightly touch the foot to the wall, but keep the other leg straight and in line with the torso. Do not place both feet against the wall or the torso will deviate from the center line. Stay for ten to twenty-five breaths, then return to the prepare position and come all the way down. Rest in Balasana for five breaths.

Try Ardha Pincha Mayurasana and Makara Adho Mukha Svanasana as alternatives to build strength if the neck is not yet prepared for weight bearing.

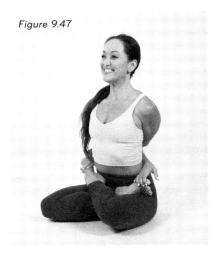

Figure 9.47

Baddha Padmasana (Bound Lotus Pose)

CHAIR VARIATION

Sit in the chair and bring the hands around the back to gently clasp the elbows. Separate the legs to facilitate a gentle rotation of the hips. Engage the pelvic floor, and lift the ribs away from the hips to support the spine. Internally rotate the shoulders to maximize the space in the shoulder joints (see fig. 9.48). Gaze toward the nose. Stay for ten breaths.

FLOOR VARIATION

Use a strap to bring the binding action closer to the hands. If Padmasana is accessible but the hands are not yet ready to bind the pose, use a strap. Sitting in Padmasana, engage the feet and wrap a strap around the insteps. Cross the arms around the back, starting with the left arm. Hold the strap firmly. Inhale and engage the muscles of the pelvic floor, draw the muscles of the lower abdomen in and up along the front of the body, lift the ribs away from the hips, internally rotate the shoulders, and engage the back muscles (see fig. 9.49).

If Padmasana is not accessible, then fold the legs into a comfortable cross-legged position and wrap a strap around the pelvis to support the same movement (see fig. 9.50). Gaze toward the nose. Stay for ten breaths.

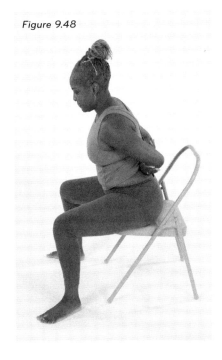

Figure 9.48

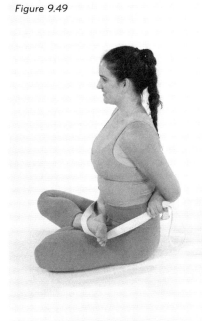

Figure 9.49

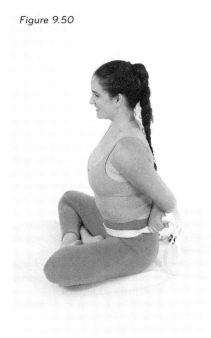

Figure 9.50

Yoga Mudra

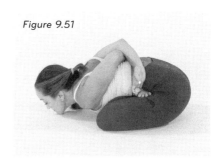
Figure 9.51

CHAIR VARIATION

Continuing directly from Baddha Padmasana, fold the torso gently forward over the hips. Pivot inside the hip joints and stabilize the legs. Maintain the position of the arms and shoulders (see fig. 9.52). Gaze toward the nose. Stay for ten breaths.

FLOOR VARIATION

Continuing directly from Baddha Padmasana, fold gently forward. Try placing the head on a block and elevating the hips to make the seated pose and the forward fold more comfortable (see fig. 9.53). Gaze toward the nose. Stay for ten breaths.

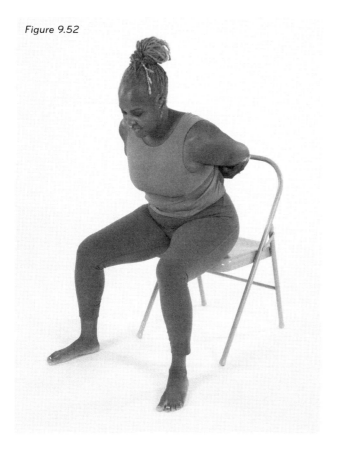
Figure 9.52

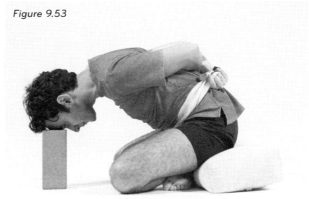
Figure 9.53

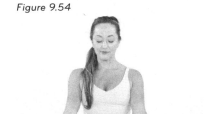
Figure 9.54

Padmasana (Full Lotus Pose)

CHAIR VARIATION

Continuing directly from Yoga Mudra, inhale and return to an upright position. Allow the hips to externally rotate slightly toward a forty-five-degree angle, and sit forward into the front of the hip joints. Maintain the activation of the pelvic floor and orient toward the center line of the body. Gently drop the head and extend the arms straight out to the knees. Place the hands in Jnana Mudra, the symbol of Divine knowledge. Press the tips of each thumb and index finger together, and extend and bring together the other three fingers (see fig. 9.55). Gaze toward the nose. Stay for ten breaths.

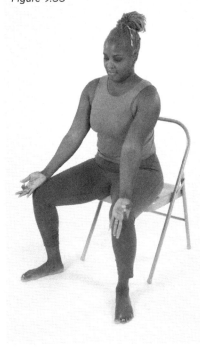
Figure 9.55

FLOOR VARIATION

Continuing directly from Yoga Mudra, return to seated. Working from a simple cross-legged position, maintain the activation of the pelvic floor and orient toward the center line of the body. Gently drop the head and extend the arms straight out to the knees. Place the hands in Jnana Mudra, the symbol of Divine knowledge. Press the tip of each thumb and index finger together, and extend and bring together the other three fingers (see fig. 9.56). If necessary, elevate the hips on a bolster or blanket to relieve pressure on the knees (see fig. 9.57). Gaze toward the nose. Stay for ten breaths.

OTHER OPTIONS

Explore Ardha Padmasana. Externally rotate the right hip joint and place the right foot along the left hip crease. If the bent knee needs support, consider placing a block under it or elevating the hips to make the hip rotation more accessible. Fold the left foot under the right thigh. Shift forward toward the front of the hip joints; if necessary, elevate the hips on a blanket to relieve pressure on the knees (see fig. 9.58). Consider switching the legs each day to work the pose equally on both sides. Gaze toward the nose. Stay for ten breaths.

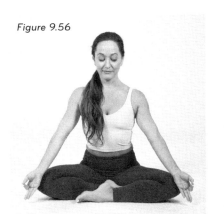
Figure 9.56

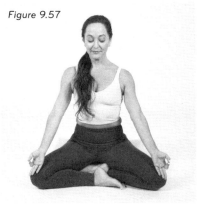
Figure 9.57

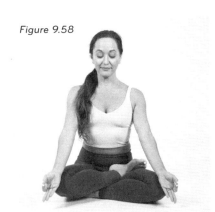
Figure 9.58

Uttplutih (Sprung Up)

CHAIR VARIATION

There are a few different ways to explore adaptations of this powerful lift. If the wrists are sore, try lifting and folding the legs into the torso and extending the arms. This can be done from the chair, the floor, a sofa, or a bed. Activate the muscles of the pelvic floor, rotate the tailbone under, and fold the ribs and hips toward each other. Curl the torso into a deep spinal flexion, then engage the muscles of the abdomen (see figs. 9.60 and 9.61). This is a great option for students who are practicing the reclining variations of the previous poses. Gaze toward the nose. Stay for ten breaths.

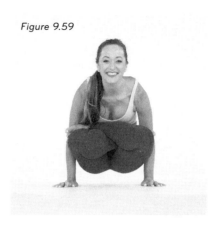

Figure 9.59

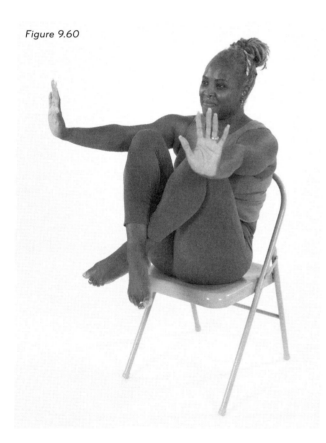

Figure 9.60

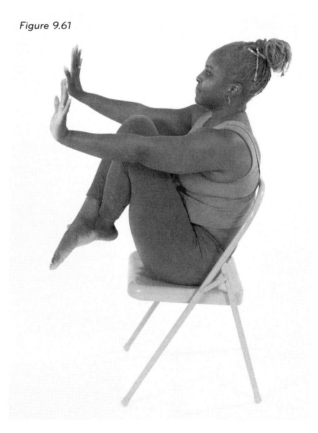

Figure 9.61

For a more ambitious use of the chair, place two chairs of equal height next to each other slightly wider than hip-width apart. Step forward toward the front of the chairs. Place the hands on the upper inner edge of the seats. Activate the muscles of the pelvic floor, rotate the tailbone under, and fold the ribs and hips toward each other. Curl the torso into a deep spinal flexion, then engage the muscles of the abdomen. Inhale and firm the shoulder girdle, press down into the hands, grip the chair, and transfer weight from the feet into the strength of the torso and arms. Slowly lift the feet off the floor (see fig. 9.62). If the feet do not lift easily, try placing them on a block or small stool and lift from there (see fig. 9.63). Gaze toward the nose. Stay for ten breaths.

Figure 9.62

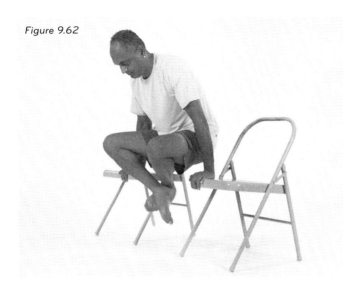

Figure 9.63

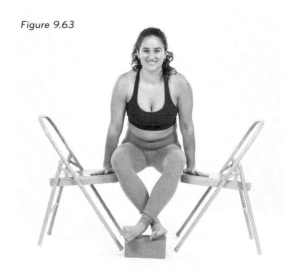

FLOOR VARIATION

Use blocks to make the lifting action more accessible. Sit in Padmasana. Place two blocks shoulder-width apart, slightly in front of the hips. Lift the lotus legs into the chest and fold the thighs close to the body. Tuck the tailbone under and work into a spinal flexion. Draw the ribs down toward the hips, engage the front of the body, and prepare the shoulder girdle for weight bearing. Inhale to root down into the hands, pitch the shoulders slightly forward, and send the hips back (fig 9.64). Avoid hooking the feet on the arms or behind the forearms. Instead, focus on maintaining the knees at the same height as the hips or higher by using the strength of the core, legs, and shoulders. The whole body is involved in this pose with a high level of activation.

If Padmasana is not accessible yet, try the lift with crossed legs (see fig. 9.65). Do not attempt the lift in any variation of Ardha Padmasana. The pressure on the core muscles and hips is not evenly distributed and can cause disruptions to the inner work of the pose. Stay for ten breaths, then return to seated.

Figure 9.64

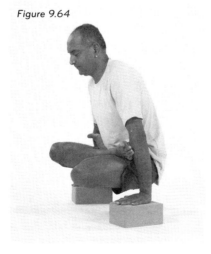

Figure 9.65

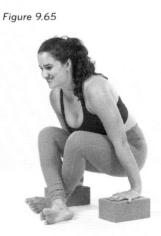

Savasana (Corpse Pose)

CHAIR VARIATION

Elevating the feet can be helpful to relieve lower back pain and pressure. Start off in a reclining position, and scoot the hips close the chair. Inhale and lift the legs onto the seat. Place the hands anywhere that is comfortable, perhaps on the abdomen (see fig. 9.67). Close the eyes. Stay for five minutes or longer.

Try finding rest seated on the chair if getting up from and down to a reclining position is not advisable. Place a bolster along the backrest of the chair. Slide the hips back so the bolster fully supports the body. Wrap a thick blanket around the neck and shoulders to support the head. Place the hands along the thighs and release the body. Close the eyes. Stay for five minutes or longer.

FLOOR VARIATION

Lie on the floor in a reclining position. Place a bolster under the backs of the knees and allow the legs to rest over the bolster. Gently roll the shoulder blades down the back. Angle the arms and legs out in a gentle external rotation. Close the eyes (see fig. 9.69). Relax the breath and bandhas. Stay for five minutes or longer.

Figure 9.66

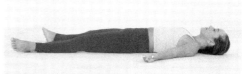

Figure 9.67

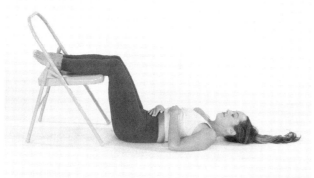

Figure 9.68

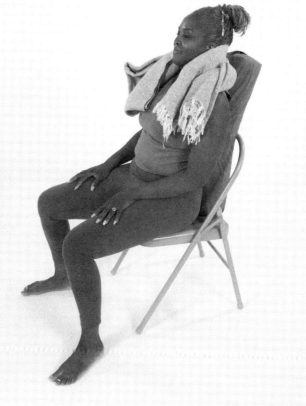

Figure 9.69

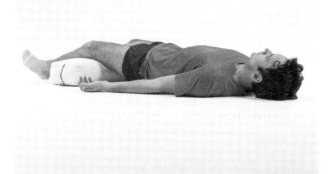

Invocations

OPENING PRAYER

ॐ

वन्दे गुरूनं चरणारविन्दे सन्दर्शित स्वात्म सुखाव बोधे
निः श्रेयसे जङ्गलिकायमाने संसार हाला हल मोहशांत्यै
आबाहु पुरुषकारं शंखचक्रासि धारिणम्
सहस्र शिरसं शवेतं प्रणमामि पतञ्जलिम

oṃ

vande gurūṇaṃ caraṇāravinde sandarśita svātma sukhāva bodhe |
niḥ śreyase jaṅgalikāyamāne saṃsāra hālā hala mohaśāntyai ||

ābāhu puruṣakāraṃ śaṅkhacakrāsi dhāriṇam |
sahasra śirasaṃ śvetaṃ praṇamāmi patañjalim ||

I bow to the lotus feet of the Gurus
The awakening happiness of one's own Self revealed,
Beyond better, acting like the Jungle physician,
Pacifying delusion, the poison of Samsara.

Taking the form of a man to the shoulders,
Holding a conch, a discus, and a sword,
One thousand heads white,
To Patanjali, I salute.

CLOSING PRAYER

ॐ

स्वस्तिप्रजाभ्यः परिपालयंतां न्यायेन मार्गेण महीं महीशाः

गोब्राह्मणेभ्यः शुभमस्तु नित्यं लोकाः समस्ताः सुखिनो भवन्तु

ॐ शान्तिः शान्तिः शान्तिः

oṃ

svastiprajābhyaḥ paripālayantāṃ nyāyena mārgeṇa mahiṃ mahiśāḥ |
gobrāhmanebhyaḥ śubhamastu nityaṃ lokāḥ samastāḥ sukhino bhavantu ||
oṃ śāntiḥ śāntiḥ śāntiḥ

May all be well with humankind.
May the leaders of the earth protect in every way by keeping to the right path.

May there be goodness for those who know the earth to be sacred.
May all the worlds be happy.

Glossary

AHIMSA Translated as "nonviolence"; the first of the yamas on the eight-limbed path of Ashtanga Yoga.

ASHTANGA YOGA The eight-limbed path of yoga devised by Patanjali; more specifically the system of yoga propagated by the late K. Pattabhi Jois that combines Patanjali's Yoga Sutras, the classical Hatha Yoga poses, and the philosophy of the Bhagavad Gita into a total system of spiritual transformation.

BANDHA Translated as "lock," referring to the three energetic locks in the body—*mula bandha* (root lock), *uddiyana bandha* (abdominal lock), and *jalandhara bandha* (throat lock).

BHAGAVAD GITA A key selection from the Mahabharata epic in which, on the eve of the great battle of Kurukhsetra, Krishna (as the avatar of God) gives the warrior prince Arjuna the teaching of yoga, sometimes given the status of an Upanishad.

BRAHMAN The one singular universal divinity, the supreme God.

CHAKRAS Translated as "wheels," the energy centers along the subtle body. There are seven main chakras in the human energy system, starting at the base of the spine and ending at the top of the head.

GUNA Translated as "strand" or "chord," referring to the three gunas (sattva, rajas, tamas) in which prakriti takes manifestation.

HATHA YOGA PRADIPIKA Classical Hatha Yoga text written approximately five hundred years ago that contains key teachings on asana, pranayama, bandhas, and other yogic practices.

MAHABHARATA The longest Sanskrit epic poem chronicling the battle between the evil Kauravas and the good Pandavas; it contains the yogic teaching of the Bhagavad Gita.

MYSORE STYLE The style of Ashtanga Yoga practice named after the city of Mysore in South India where K. Pattabhi Jois lived, in which students memorize the poses and go at their own pace, awaiting help from the teacher only when necessary.

NADI Energy channels running through the subtle body that yoga purifies. Seventy-two thousand are mentioned in classical Hatha Yoga texts.

NADI SHODHANA Translated as "nadi or nerve cleansing"; associated with both the Intermediate Series of Ashtanga Yoga and alternate nostril breathing exercises.

PRAKRITI Nature, the eternally changeable manifest world of mind and matter, comprising the three gunas.

PRANAYAMA Breathing exercises that purify the body in classical yogic practice; also the fourth limb of the eight-limbed path of Ashtanga Yoga in Patanjali's Yoga Sutras.

PURUSHA The eternal, deathless, changeless Self in traditional yoga philosophy, sometimes taken to mean the individual soul or the universal soul.

RISHI Translated as "seer"; usually taken to mean the seer who originally received the Vedas.

SAMSKARA Repetitive behavioral and thought patterns that take root within the citta.

SATTVA One of the three gunas, associated with peace, harmony, and balance.

SATYA Translated as "true essence"; the second of the yamas listed in Patanjali's Yoga Sutras.

SUBTLE BODY The body composed of subtle sensations that are often imperceptible to the untrained mind.

TAPAS Translated as "heat"; the third of the niyamas and the first component of Kriya Yoga in Patanjali's Yoga Sutras. Associated with the fire of purification cultivated in Ashtanga Yoga.

VINYASA The coordination of breath with movement that is the foundation of the Ashtanga Yoga method; the system of counting each movement in the yoga practice with a Sanskrit number.

YOGA CHIKITSA Yoga therapy, also known as the Primary Series of Ashtanga Yoga as taught by K. Pattabhi Jois.

About the Author

KINO MACGREGOR is a lifelong spiritual seeker, a Miami native who is happiest on the beach with a fresh coconut. She is the founder of Omstars—the world's first yoga TV network, where you can practice with Kino live (www.omstars.com)—and the cofounder of Miami Yoga Garage, where you can find her teaching in person with her husband, Tim Feldmann. With over one million followers on Instagram and over eight hundred thousand subscribers on YouTube and Facebook, Kino's message of spiritual strength reaches people all over the world. Sought after worldwide as a yoga expert for classes, workshops, retreats, and trainings, she is an inspirational speaker, the author of multiple books, a podcaster, and a teacher of teachers.

Yoga for Kino is a way of life founded on a firm commitment to the moral and ethical precepts of truth, nonviolence, and love. With over twenty-five years of dedicated personal practice in both Ashtanga Yoga and Vipassana meditation, Kino believes in making the tools of traditional yoga accessible for all different sizes, shapes, ethnicities, and ages. Yoga is more than the poses, and she believes we must take the lessons learned off the mat into real life.